Paying the Doctor

Paying the Doctor

HEALTH POLICY AND PHYSICIAN REIMBURSEMENT

EDITED BY

Jonathan D. Moreno

AUBURN HOUSE

NEW YORK • WESTPORT, CONNECTICUT • LONDON

Library of Congress Cataloging-in-Publication Data

Paying the doctor : health policy and physician reimbursement / edited
  by Jonathan D. Moreno.
       p.   cm
    Includes index.
    ISBN 0-86569-006-5 (lib. bdg. : alk. paper)
    1. Medical fees--United States. 2. Medicare. 3. Medicaid.
  I. Moreno, Jonathan D.
R728.5.P37 1991
331.2'81362173'0973--dc20   90-37837

British Library Cataloguing in Publication Data is available.

Library of Congress Catalog Card Number: 90–37837
ISBN: 0-86569-006-5

First published in 1991

Auburn House, 88 Post Road West, Westport, CT 06881
An imprint of Greenwood Publishing Group, Inc.

Printed in the United States of America

∞

The paper used in this book complies with the
Permanent Paper Standard issued by the National
Information Standards Organization (Z39.48-1984).

10 9 8 7 6 5 4 3 2 1

Contents

Acknowledgments

The editor expresses his gratitude to Dick Riegelman, who conceived of this book and whose energy and creativity potently combined to help move this project through the usual obstacles. Maureen Flaherty provided her sense of administrative orderliness in helping the editor keep track of mechanical matters. Special thanks to Greg Pawlson and the Department of Health Care Sciences at The George Washington University for their continuing commitment to multidisciplinary studies of the health care system. I am particularly grateful to Maxine Mantell and Annette Bishop, who assisted with several thankless last minute editorial jobs.

Finally, thanks to all the participants in this project, who tolerated a stream of memoranda from the editor—and seem even to have read some of them!

Introduction

Jonathan D. Moreno

About sixty years ago, my father accepted a position as the medical officer of a small town outside Vienna. Because the job included a house provided by the state, and because he possessed the idealism of a newly minted physician, he did not charge the poorer peasant farmers whom he treated. One day there came a knock on his door. Upon opening it, he saw that an old man who had been his patient some months before had returned, this time accompanied by a young woman who appeared to be about fifteen or sixteen years old. "Doctor Moreno," the old man said, "you cured me of a stomach disorder that plagued me for years, and I have been thinking about how to express my gratitude. Here is my daughter. She has no husband, and you should have a wife. Please, take her with my thanks."

My father declined the offer, as far as I know.

The specific problems associated with physician reimbursement have changed quite a bit since the time this incident took place, but in a broad, philosophical sense it illustrates a reason the entire subject makes many of us uneasy. For although we are accustomed to think about compensating people for the goods they produce or the services they provide, there are some things that others can do for us for which the idea of payment seems somehow incongruous. Particularly in the sphere of health care, how can one measure the value of being healed (literally, being made whole) when one is at one's most vulnerable? How can this be reduced to reimbursable terms? Competing with this philosophical uneasiness is an economic realism that should not be dismissed as crass: Of course, in an abstract sense no product or service, including health care, has a specific value. Only in the marketplace do such measures make sense; in that context all items can be priced.

Strictly speaking, these two points of view are quite compatible, for one can always accept the realities of market mechanisms while puzzling about the more general significance of health care for human life. Yet the tension between the strangeness of placing a market value on health care and the trivial familiarity of this process seems to stand in the background of much of the public debate about this matter. Thus, a familiar issue is what the proper role of the health care provider should be in setting rates for his or her own compensation: Considering the inherent conflict of interest in fee-for-service medicine, should that be considered the ideal? Rather, if care-givers are to be reimbursed in a "cost conscious" fashion, how can the patient be protected, and from what? Regardless of the choices made, what constraints does the marketplace impose on patients, providers, managers, and legislators?

We have chosen to begin this volume on physician reimbursement by explicitly addressing these questions, which will surface again and again in subsequent chapters. Though it is generally agreed that no systematic study of the area can proceed without an understanding of the issues that have been mentioned, we know of no other effort both to engage them and to weigh the subtle options that health care financing involves. Also critical in this complex policy picture are the diverse roles of primary care physicians, specialists, and allied health professionals, viewpoints that are incorporated in this volume. Finally, we have included thorough historical, political, and structural analyses of the Medicare system as the most recent example of deliberate reform of reimbursement practices in the United States. Introductions to the parts are provided to help orient the reader to the specific concerns they contain as well as to provide continuity and perspective. The conclusion describes the major provisions of the payment system that will be implemented in 1992 and gives a blow-by-blow account of the political process that led finally to this legislation.

A volume of this scope, yet directed at such a specific subject, would be impossible without contributors who specialize in the dynamics of the health care system and yet who have backgrounds in an exceptionally broad range of disciplines. It was serendipitous that a large number of George Washington University faculty members from various academic departments were interested in physician reimbursement and were prepared to join forces in such a study: physicians and other health care providers, policy analysts, economists, health care administrators, historians, and philosophers. The goal was to create a volume nontechnical enough to serve as an introduction to the subject for practicing physicians and other health care professionals, as well as one sophisticated enough to be of interest to researchers in the field. Further, it is hoped that these efforts will be of persistent value over the next few years, even as the specifics of physician payment reform continue to take shape.

Part I
Analyzing the Issues

To help the reader gain a grasp of a complex and highly specialized area, we begin with a series of studies that both describe and apply various frameworks for analyzing physician payment. In reality, ethics, economics, and quality assurance are of course closely intertwined, but it is helpful to understand their perspectives separately at first. Later chapters will draw them together again.

The idea of a profession is one that we frequently call on, especially in conversations about responsibility and autonomy, but often without being very clear about what specifically the idea of professionalism entails. Gary Crum assesses a number of different efforts to identify the elements of a profession before settling on his list, an important item on which is the notion of a calling. From this angle he shows exactly what a fundamental challenge the entire subject of reimbursement presents to the medical profession, one that reaches beyond specific ethical issues to the very way in which physicians understand themselves and what they do.

Jacqueline J. Glover and Gail J. Povar carry this theme into their focus on the contemporary environment of physician reimbursement in any industrialized economy, one that is characterized by cost-consciousness. Taking as their point of departure the recent concept of the physician as a gatekeeper charged partly with guarding the appropriate use of valuable health care resources, Glover and Povar articulate and examine critically the proposition that physicians should be held at least partly responsible for the just allocation of health care resources. They are skeptical of the traditional notion that the doctor who sees him- or herself as simply an advocate for the particular presenting patient is on safe moral ground.

Quality assurance is still too often regarded as a merely mechanical activity in our health care institutions, but as pressures for reform of the system continue, it seems wise to appreciate its potentially crucial role in the protection of patients' best interests. Molla Donaldson surveys the history and concept of quality assurance, highlighting the question of how quality can be subjected to measurement. If changes in the health care system are to benefit patients, then the process of change must not proceed in ignorance of the sorts of incentives for physicians that at least will not impede this goal.

While the literature on physician reimbursement has paid a great deal of attention to the financing of physician payment, the underlying relevant economic theory vastly enriches our understanding of the financial options. Proceeding from an exposition of the market system, Mary Ann Baily notes the limitations of that model as it applies to health care services. Aspects of all three of the previous chapters reappear as Baily offers a set of remedies that complements several of the most frequently suggested financial alternatives. But no matter which alternatives are chosen, Baily warns, financial incentives to physicians alone will probably not result in a delivery system that most people will find acceptable.

In reaching this conclusion by way of economic theory, Baily effectively reminds us of the multifactorial nature of our topic, that it is too often reduced to financing issues alone. Thus, our success in this volume is closely related to our ability to keep many different balls in the air. We have introduced a few in this part and will have to engage health services administration, history, and politics later in the book. But perhaps the present themes will keep us busy enough in this first part.

1

Professionalism and Physician Reimbursement

Gary Crum

The medical vocation is one of the classic professional groups, as are the law, clergy, and military. As a profession the medical vocation has been granted certain privileges by society: high pay, professional powers (e.g., prescription control), and self-policing (e.g., control of licensure and control of entry into professional schooling, the so-called gatekeeping control).

This chapter begins with an examination of the various factors that distinguish professions from other vocations and is followed by a discussion of how the choice of payment mechanism—whether by salary or by fee-for-service—can affect the nature of the medical profession. The special ethical questions raised by independent practice associations with their mix of prepayment and fee-for-service payment mechanisms will not be addressed.[1] The question this chapter does seek to answer is a normative one: How *ought* the doctor to be paid, from the perspective of medical professionalism and the profession's advantages and disadvantages to society?

THE QUALITIES OF A PROFESSION AND PROFESSIONAL CALLING

Wilbert Moore, like virtually all writers on this topic, has noted the difficulties associated with defining professionalism. He developed a list of criteria with a variety of subscales and values and cautioned against any effort to draw hard and fast lines between true and false professions. His criteria for professionalism were these: (1) The profession is an occupation that serves as the principal source of income, (2) it involves a calling—what he defined as "an enduring set of normative and behavioral expectations," (3) it requires education that is difficult and/or lengthy, (4) it has a service orientation, and (5) it enjoys a certain amount of autonomy in its practice.[2]

Elliott Krause[3] has taken a different look at the professions. Beginning with the topic of the division of labor in society, he investigated such questions as whether or not the occupation group could immediately paralyze society by refusing to work. He noted that the importance of the job to society and the need for lengthy education for the job were important considerations in determining where society ranks various jobs on its division-of-labor scale.

A key point for Krause was the requirement that professions not only wield special intellectual abilities, but also wield these abilities in "crisis-relevant" functions such as "health, liberty, and property, the meaning of existence, and national self-defense" (p. 75). He also noted the importance to the concept of profession of other attributes—namely, the paternalistic role of the professional in relation to his/her client, self-regulation, intra-professional culture, and a self-defined and enforced code of ethics.

John Cullen[4] reviewed fourteen different literature sources for the best definition of profession. From these sources he found ten attributes of professions that were most commonly mentioned: an organized and complex occupation, long training, a code of ethics, person-oriented, licensed, altruistic service, high income and prestige, and self-employment.

Michael Bayles[5] suggested three features that he felt were "necessary" attributes for every true profession and three additional features that were common attributes, though not uniformly required. The first of his three necessary features was extensive training. Bayles believed that an advanced college degree was a prerequisite for professional status. His second necessary feature, a significant intellectual component, was related to the first feature. The third necessary feature he believed to be important service to society. He noted that the increase in the number of professionals in modern society might be due mainly to the increasing complexity of society and society's attendant need for skilled, organized services.

Bayles' common, but not necessary, features of professions were certification/licensing, organization or members, and autonomy. He further discussed a two-category taxonomy for professions—those with clients (e.g., law and medicine) and those without (e.g., teaching and journalism). He categorized those with clients as consulting professions and those without clients as scholarly professions.[6]

The author's preference for a list of the necessary prerequisites that must be met before a vocation becomes a true profession results in inclusion of the three mentioned by Bayles, but with a slightly different emphasis.[7] Two of Bayles' features—extensive training and intellectual expertise—it seems could be easily merged into educational attainment, since the line between being able to complete training successfully and having intelligence seems too thin to justify two separate categories. In regard to Bayles' necessary feature of important service to society, it seems that the concept of calling that was discussed by Moore might be more appropriate. Also, Cullen's finding of the attribute of altruism in some of the profession definitions he researched helps to support the idea that calling should be considered one of the required characteristics of professions—a characteristic that not only refers to the profession's being important to society, but also refers more specifically to a particular view of the common good. A profession's calling is not only to be something desired by a particular society; it should address universal needs and values that represent society's highest ideals and increase its internal cohesiveness.

The term *calling* is historically reserved for those in the clergy—that is, as a divine summons to undertake some selfless task—but with only slight alteration it can be used to refer to the profession's chief and highest motives for existing and for being granted certain privileges by the society that it serves. For the lawyer, it is a calling to justice; for the military officer, it is a calling to national security; and for the medical profession, it is a calling to healing or health care. Only such a motive for the profession's members could give normative weight to the profession's claims to privileges over and above those granted the average member of society. By the same token, as a profession moves away from its calling, it risks becoming a bane rather than a boon to the society that granted it special status among the vocations.

In regard to the characteristic of educational attainment, it is by a proper understanding of the role of the profession's calling that professional education can be seen in its proper light. Krause's comments about an intra-professional culture can be translated as a need for the professions to educate new members in the calling of the vocation, and the code of ethics can be translated as a key tool for expressing the primary professional behaviors and cultural values that the new members must internalize successfully during their educational experience. The profession cannot fail to exercise gatekeeping restrictions using standards based on both factual educational attainment and intraprofessional culture assimilation. Otherwise, persons with little dedication to the public's good would find themselves representing the profession in that society. This is more than a violation of public trust; it is also a dire risk to the acceptability of that profession by the society.

PROFESSIONAL EFFECTS OF MOVING TOWARD SALARIED PHYSICIANS

Bayles, in summarizing Eliot Freidson's work, has made the following statement in regard to the above-mentioned difference between consulting professions and scholarly professions:

The consulting professions, such as law, medicine, and architecture, have traditionally practiced on a fee-for-service basis with a personal, individual relationship between client and professional. A consulting professional (or a professional in a

consulting role) acts primarily in behalf of an individual client. A scholarly professional, such as a college teacher or scientific researcher, usually has many clients at
the same time (students) or no personal client (jobs assigned by superiors in a
corporation). A scholarly professional usually works for a salary rather than as an
entrepreneur who depends on attracting individual clients. . . . These differences between the roles of consulting and scholarly professionals are crucial in defining the
kinds of ethical problems each confronts.[8]

More than 40 percent of all physicians under thirty-five are currently
being paid by salary, a much higher percentage than is observed among
older physicians, according to Arnold Relman.[9] Another factor might be
the increased numbers of physicians who are being graduated each year. As
David Mechanic has noted, "Doctors will no longer have the ability to resist
administrative and managerial pressures as they did when they were in short
supply" (p. 11).[10] Others have listed some additional reasons for the changing picture.[11, 12, 13]

As the medical profession moves from a fee-for-service, consulting profession to a salaried, scholarly profession, several ramifications will require a
rethinking of the proper role of the physician in society. Among the advantages that can accrue when any profession moves from a fee-for-service
to a salaried arrangement is the opportunity for more altruism, according
to Bayles. This is because of the removal of any financial conflicts of interest
that might come into play in the method by which the professionals select
which patients to treat. However, if the organizations paying the physicians'
salaries place sanctions against those physicians who select clients based on
this increased altruism, this advantage of salaries would not seem likely to
be observed. The conflict of interest has only passed from the individual
physician to the corporate entity, which would in some cases be even less
predisposed to altruism than the physician who is face to face with the
suffering of his or her patients.

Another factor that affects and is encouraged by the movement to salaries
is the team approach to professionalism.[14] As the physician moves into team
and group arrangements and away from the private practice model of providing services, more evaluation by professional colleagues (and other organizational personnel) and more specialization occur. The causes and
results are mixed, with specialization driving a need for team medicine and
with team development encouraging divisions of labor for economic efficiencies. The medical profession has thus far been able to enjoy the advantages of specialization without losing prestige and autonomy because the
medical profession has required that even specialists must complete the
general practitioner curriculum first. In engineering, for example, the training of specialists (e.g., chemical or aerospace engineers) does not follow so
stringent a course.

There may be a push to permit specialists to bypass much of the general practitioner training as medicine is more and more bureaucratized, in order to shorten the training time for specialists and make them more quickly available to the medical financial enterprise. This would remove much of the entrepreneurial aspects of medicine by denying specialists the option of practicing medicine on their own, as well as by reducing the specialists' comprehensive understanding of disease that is beneficial when treating patients with more than one neatly categorized disease. However, a change from the current practice of giving all physicians a general practitioner's training does not seem to be a likely occurrence in the near future.

A change much more likely to take place as medicine moves from a client-centered profession to a scholarly profession will be the alteration of the calling of the profession. As decisions are being influenced more and more by organizational priorities and financial solvency, and as the hiring of physicians and the maintenance of their privileges are increasingly tied to corporate income projections and economies of scale, the healing calling of the medical profession will take on an added dimension. The calling will become a calling toward efficient healing—or even to efficiency in healing, where the concept of organizational and economic efficiencies is the driving consideration and healing is only the dimension in which efficiency happens to be pursued.

One result of this altered calling will be a loss of the physician's ability to view the patient as solely an individual. Even though the patient might have previously had his or her individual goals relegated to a minority status in the mind of the physician when the public health was threatened by the patient's behavior, the physician would not typically have been considering the public wealth. The physician-patient relationship must undergo an important change insofar as the public wealth or the organizational wealth becomes a factor in the decisions that the physician makes for an individual patient. The physician becomes an agent for two groups that may be in an adversarial position, and the healing calling is now at odds with the organizational efficiency calling.

For example, suppose an elderly male patient presents himself with a condition that could be treated by an expensive new procedure that has only recently gone beyond the research stage. His physician is aware of the new procedure, but it would be extremely expensive to provide this procedure to the patient. The health maintenance organization (HMO) for which the physician works has been encouraging physicians to keep unnecessary admissions to the HMO's hospital down and has been running in the red for the last three years. Instead of recommending the new procedure, the physician recommends a traditional approach, using a drug that even then the physician does not think would be as good for the patient as a much more expensive, and slightly more effective, drug that is not on the drug formulary of the HMO. In this situation a fee-for-service physician might have treated the patient more effectively from a healing standpoint, but certainly less efficiently from a financial viewpoint.

This situation need not be a loss to patients as a group even though this individual patient might suffer. For example, if the patient's condition does not worsen *and* cause additional HMO expenses, the aggregate benefit to HMO patients might be more money to keep an HMO solvent and operating in an area where no accessible alternative treatment setting is available. If the HMO has three more years of operating in the red, the patient may find that the only local health service will go bankrupt and decrease his health service access. Thus, as patient care is made more efficient, even at the cost to an individual patient's healing, the healing goal may become more sure for patients as a whole within the community. Here the physician has adopted efficiency as a new wrinkle on the healing calling, but is requiring that the economic aspects of efficiency be designed still with patients as a group in mind. In the words of Gail Povar and Jonathan Moreno, "[i]t is not unreasonable to argue that the institution and its physicians have an obligation to act as advocates for the community of patients who participate in the [HMO] program, and not only for the individual patient" (p. 422).[1] The worst case scenario might be when the physician adopts efficiency in order to further a goal other than even indirect healing. If the goal that requires reducing the individual-centeredness and professional autonomy of physicians is to increase the value of a for-profit corporation's stocks, or to purchase a new television set for the corporation president's yacht, then the medical profession has placed efficiency and economic concerns before healing. Healing becomes another means to make money, like selling shoes or corn futures. Health care becomes another potentially lucrative market, rather than a value held in high esteem by society.

One final point to be discussed is the vulnerable nature of the sick individual. This individual is often dependent on the healing skill of his or her physician for life itself. Such a client is more vulnerable than any other professional's client, save the lawyer's client who is charged with a capital crime. As a physician, Stanley Troup, has stated:

If the patient cannot count on his or her interests being held paramount by the physician, it is unlikely that proper care can follow. Recommendations from the physician, whether in terms of diagnosis or proposed treatment, are less likely to be accepted and followed. Even if they are accepted and followed, the toll on the patient in terms of uncertainty, fear, and foreboding will be enormous (p. 10).[15]

It is at this point that the calling of the medical profession must be most unshakable. It is here that society perhaps has the greatest reason to grant privilege and autonomy for the medical profession, and it is here that the medical profession can cause the greatest damage to society when responsibilities for healing are made secondary. The patient facing death, with an acute or a chronic illness, gains comfort in just knowing that the physician is his or her advocate against this universal enemy, this primeval fear.

Insofar as society gives up this personal doctor-patient healing relationship for a group healing relationship—let alone for a financially driven relationship—then society has decreased one of its most rudimentary services to its members. The loss of this service can perhaps be adequately justified by pointing to greater numbers of statistical lives saved by the profession when groups of patients are considered over individual patients, but it seems plain that the loss ought not to be considered acceptable when it is balanced with dollars rather than lives. (At least one court has also said that the physician must legally take responsibility for patient care decisions even when such decisions are actively opposed by the third-party payer involved in the case— *Wickline v. California.*[16])

In closing, I will relate a personal anecdote. During the early 1970s I worked as a governmental health planner for the Commonwealth of Kentucky. Under the health-planning programs then in effect, I was always seeking physicians to serve on statewide planning committees. The best such physicians, in my mind, were those who could look at the big health policy picture and who did not think that centralized planning for hospitals and clinics was an encroachment on the profession of medicine. With a few such physicians, and a large group of consumers, I think that I helped the state government to develop a more efficient and accessible health care system, particularly in regard to service to rural areas. However, even at that time, I would never seek out this same type of physician for my personal care. I wanted a physician who was my personal advocate for health when I was facing dire illness. No matter how minor the advantage, I wanted every test that might prevent unnecessary suffering or death—I wanted state-of-the-art medicine no matter what the cost.

I could not legally demand that medical care of society if I did not have the resources to pay for it; but I wanted and needed an expert advocate who could tell me what was best for me with nothing that was potentially helpful held back. If there was a million dollar operation available in Geneva, I wanted to know about it.

That was the professional advice I desired, physically, mentally, and socially, when I was sick. I feel even more strongly today that that is the ideal type of physician needed by society. When we lose access to the physician who is oriented to individual healing, we had better be getting an excellent group healing consolation prize. Otherwise, we have traded our well-being for a mess of potage.

As the number of salaried physicians increases in relation to the number of physicians being paid by their individual clients, the medical profession will move from one subtype of profession to another. We may find that the advantages of this move are the opportunity for more altruism in the absence of pecuniary motivations on the part of the physician and the development of a more accessible and equitable health care system; or we may find that altruism is reduced as the calling of the physician becomes more and more oriented to the organization paying his or her salary and less and less autonomous in regard to putting the individual patient first. The net advantage or disadvantage that results will to a large part be determined by the medical profession's ability to maintain the privileges gained by the profession in regard to such elements as prescription writing, medical school gatekeeping, and self-policing, and especially by the willingness of the profession to make its own values and code of ethics a source of no-compromise relationships with its local employers. As Relman has noted concerning a physician's responsibility as his or her patients' advocate, "[t]he economic interests of an employer should not be permitted to interfere with a physician's ability to meet that basic responsibility."[9] The profession will in effect have given up its autonomy if the payers of the profession's salaries are able to alter substantially the healing decisions of individual professionals who are trying to act in the best interests of individual patients. It will have ceased to be a profession, or will at least have become a so-called scholarly profession driven by two sometimes antagonistic callings, healing and organizational efficiency, rather than by just the calling to heal.

If the calling to efficiency is at least added in a subsidiary role to the calling to heal, patients may see their medical bills go down and their access to some health care services improved, at the expense of not having quite as confidential and dedicated an advocate at the point of their life when they are most vulnerable. This would be an important change in the medical profession, but not as great as if the calling to efficiency came to dominate the calling to heal. The crucial point for the profession itself will come when it finally decides, overtly or by default, whether or not the constraints of efficiency installed by the organization paying physicians' salaries must be oriented, at least indirectly, to patient health concerns rather than being oriented to an organization's or even society's nonhealth-related financial agenda. If medical efficiency becomes not even indirectly tied to a patient benefit, medicine will have been reconstituted as just another vocation for potential business entrepreneurs, and society will have auctioned off one of its greatest guarantees of personal security for a few dollars.

NOTES

The author would like to express his appreciation for the assistance he received from Kevin Criswell in the preparation of this chapter.

1. For a discussion of these issues, see G. Povar and J. Moreno, "Hippocrates and the Health Maintenance Organization," *Annals of Internal Medicine* 109 (1988): 419–24.

2. W. Moore, *The Professions, Roles and Rules* (New York: Russell Sage Foundation, 1970), p. 5.

3. E. Krause, *The Sociology of Occupations* (Boston: Little, Brown and Co., 1971).

4. J. Cullen, *The Structure of Professionalism: A Quantitative Examination* (New York: Petrocelli Books, 1978).

5. M. Bayles, *Professional Ethics* (Belmont, Calif.: Wadsworth, 1981).

6. Both consulting and scholarly professions are scholarly in that they require extensive education, so a better taxonomy might be to refer to them as entrepreneurial versus bureaucratic professions, individual-oriented versus group-oriented professions, or autonomous versus nonautonomous professions. Nevertheless, for the purposes of this current study, the terms *consulting* and *scholarly* will be retained.

7. G. Crum, "Professionalism and the Field of Health Planning" (Master's thesis, George Washington University, 1983).

8. E. Freidson, ed., *The Professions and Their Prospects* (Beverly Hills, Calif.: Sage, 1973), p. 9.

9. A. Relman, "Salaried Physicians and Economic Incentives," *New England Journal of Medicine* 319 (1988): 784.

10. D. Mechanic, "Physicians and Patients in Transition," *Hastings Center Report* 15 (1985): 9–12.

11. C. Gaus et al., "Contrasts in HMO and Fee-for-Service Performance," *Social Security Bulletin* 39 (1976): 3–14.

12. G. Engel and R. Hall, "The Growing Industrialization of the Professions," in E. Freidson, ed., *The Professions and Their Prospects* (Beverly Hills, Calif.: Sage, 1973).

13. L. J. Goodman and J. Swartwout, "Comparative Aspects of Medical Practice: Organizational Setting and Financial Arrangements in Four Delivery Systems," *Medical Care* 22 (1984): 255–66.

14. W. Manning et al., "A Controlled Trial of the Effect of a Pre-paid Group Practice on the Use of Services," *New England Journal of Medicine* 310 (1984): 1505–10.

15. S. Troup, "Doctor-Patient Relationship: A Covenant of Trust?" *Medical Ethics for the Physician* 3 (1988): 5, 10.

16. J. Fleetwood, "The Physician's Role in Keeping Costs Down," *Medical Ethics for the Physician* 4 (1989): 11–12.

2

The Ethics of Cost-Conscious Physician Reimbursement

Jacqueline J. Glover and Gail J. Povar

Decisions regarding patient care are inevitably influenced by decisions regarding payment. In an ideal world, we might want physicians and other providers such as hospitals to be paid for doing exactly the right thing for patients without financial incentives to provide either too much or too little care. In the real world, however, such a reimbursement scheme is clearly impossible. In fact, society uses reimbursement as a mechanism to promote other social values, such as efficiency, cost containment, and the just allocation of health care resources, which may be at odds with benefit to the individual patient.

In an effort to allocate resources wisely, physicians have been identified as gatekeepers who can be pressured, primarily through reimbursement mechanisms, to make cost-conscious decisions within a framework of advocacy for the welfare of individual patients. Such a vision of physicians as gatekeepers has ethical implications. Does the just allocation of health care resources require or forbid physician gatekeeping? Even if our concept of justice requires some form of gatekeeping, should physicians be exempt from taking on such responsibilities? Does gatekeeping violate the physician's role-specific duty to be an advocate for the welfare of individual patients?

As we consider an ethical framework within which to analyze the question of physician gatekeeping, we ought to be mindful of two important observations. First, physicians are unavoidably involved in questions of health care allocation. Even if we separate allocation decisions from special financial incentives, physicians will always be gatekeepers. They control access to much that the health care delivery system offers, from laboratory tests to prescription drugs. Indeed, doctors' decisions account for as much as 80 percent of all health care expenditures.[1] The question is really not whether physicians should be gatekeepers, but whether their obligations require them to be the kind of gatekeepers that only keep the gate open, never closed.

A second observation is that conflict of interest is inevitable. We sometimes speak as though conflict of interest is unique to the era of cost containment. In fact, reimbursement schemes such as fee-for-service may tempt physicians to provide too many services just as other schemes might pressure them to provide too few. It is not immediately obvious which is better for the patient. In any case we have historically relied on the physician's professional responsibility for the patient's welfare to counteract incentives to overutilization. The same responsibility could counteract incentives to underutilization. In fact, if physicians *do* regard the possibility of doing too little as more dangerous than the reverse, then a professional ethic of patient advocacy seems even more likely to be engaged in such situations. Yet critics point to the failure of professional responsibility to counteract either set of incentives.

Conflicts of interest have lead some to argue that physician reimbursement should be separated as much as possible from clinical decisions. In the extreme, physicians become salaried employees, without bonuses attached to utilization patterns. However, even this approach would not eliminate conflict of interest, for there would still be a tension between the welfare of the patient and the welfare of the physician's employer. Ultimately, we must acknowledge that no reimbursement scheme is going to be conflict-free. The question then is not how to *avoid* conflict of interest, but how to *minimize* it.

AN EXPANDED ETHICAL FRAMEWORK

The traditional ethical framework for medical decision making focuses on individual clinical relationships. Decisions reflect the medical expertise of the physician and the values and preferences of the patient. The physician, in this view, serves as the advocate for the well-being of the particular patient, according to the patient's own idiosyncratic understanding of well-being. The principle of justice is viewed as somehow outside of this personal medical relationship. It is assumed that a just distribution of resources results inevitably from the aggregate of personal decisions.

Such an "invisible hand" account of justice in health care is problematic, however. Justice understood as fairness would seem to require that every member of the community have access to some adequate level of health care. There are presently about 35 million Americans who have no health care insurance and therefore very limited access to services.[2] Providing them all access to even basic services would be very expensive. It is doubtful we can or ought to expand our health care spending infinitely to meet the demands of increased access for those who have none, as well as to meet those demands arising from the continual development and application of new and costly technology and from the increase in prevalence of chronic disease. Unlimited spending by some places at risk the availability of services to others.

Even if we increase health care spending, the need to allocate wisely can never be eliminated. Claiming that an unlimited allocation for health care is the only just approach is to argue that any money is better spent on health care than on any other goods that must be foregone. Human health needs are limitless, and so, too, are the possibilities for medical benefit; yet some interventions clearly offer more benefit than others. If we are to provide each member of the community adequate access to health care services, and to provide other kinds of community services as well, trade-offs are necessary. Justice would thus seem to require some modification of the individualistic framework of medical decision making. If unlimited spending by some puts at risk even the basic availability of resources for others, such spending should be limited. A more comprehensive ethical framework for medical decision making would include not only what one physician recommends and what one patient prefers, but also what the community can afford. Within such a framework, justice is not an afterthought, but an integral part of the determination of appropriate care.

Considering a Just Allocation of Resources

How should one incorporate a principle of justice into medical decision making? As described above, a principle of justice as fairness would require equal access to some adequate level of health care for all.[3] Cost containment offers one approach to promoting justice to the extent that unrestrained spending contributes to the misallocation of health care resources. But there is nothing inherent to a certain percentage of the gross national product (GNP) that will indicate whether too much, too little, or just the right amount of money is being spent on health care as compared with other community goods. Likewise, efficient use of health care dollars may increase the overall benefits achieved, but no specific ratio of cost effectiveness is necessarily *the* morally correct one.

Therefore, while efficiency and cost containment may be important, they are not moral values in themselves. What matters is the goal of increased access that they share. Certainly increased efficiency may yield benefits to patients in the form of reduced insurance costs, consumer prices, or taxes that might accompany lower health care costs generally, but such benefits cannot be assured and are not necessarily related to a fair allocation of health care resources. Cost containment and efficiency could also serve to increase the profits of investor-owned hospitals or ambulatory care centers. The relationship of such profits to patient welfare and just allocation is also unclear. Cost containment and efficiency are most justifiable when they are used to further the moral objective of equitable access. It would be unjust, therefore, to invoke cost containment as the rationale for denying access to adequate services to individuals who need them.

Additionally, the principle of justice as fairness will have something to say about the way in which trade-offs can be made. A concept of adequate health care will be difficult, at best, to implement. There will be categories of patients whose conditions are such that they cannot be improved and large amounts of resources will be necessary simply to maintain them. A concept of adequacy that excludes such patients would seem to violate a principle of justice as fairness.

Also, what counts as marginal benefit that can be foregone in the name of better alternative uses of the funds cannot depend in this system of justice on the disvaluing of such vulnerable individuals. We cannot call fair or just an allocation scheme that ignores the needs of categories of individuals, such as the elderly or the handicapped, for example. Any cost-benefit analysis must acknowledge the risk of categorically labeling the assistance offered to vulnerable patients as less beneficial than assistance offered to those who can be returned to "normalcy."

PHYSICIANS' JUSTICE-BASED OBLIGATIONS

Some would argue that it is precisely this principle of justice as fairness that would require physicians to leave the allocation of resources to other parties.[4, 5, 6, 7] Ideally, we want judgments about the distribution of social goods to be unbiased. If we also want our physicians to be as biased for each of us as possible, then they are in the worst position to make so-called objective choices. Furthermore, physician choices would idiosyncratically represent only the values of physicians. Such an idiosyncratic and narrow perspective is exactly what any principle of justice would forbid.

Additionally, what particular expertise do physicians have to allocate resources justly? Simply because physicians, and other professionals, have unique expertise in a particular field, does not mean they are qualified to make judgments on matters outside their own area of special knowledge. When it comes to allocating resources justly, trade-offs are necessary not only among medical options, but also among all social goods. Physicians are not necessarily qualified to assess the relative benefits of medicine and other social goods, such as education, for example, which is outside of their area of expertise. Additionally, physicians are likely to be biased in favor of medicine and will rank it higher than other goods, just as a teacher might rank education higher, or a soldier, defense. Such an argument would provide the basis for a claim that physicians cannot be the *only* gatekeepers in society, but must join with other community representatives in balancing all social goods in a just allocation scheme. However, some critics would go further to argue that physicians cannot be negative gatekeepers at all.

In their view, physicians should be exempt from obligations to distributive justice because it would compromise their role as patient advocate.

PHYSICIANS' OBLIGATIONS AS ADVOCATES

At the center of the controversy over physician gatekeeping is concern for the preservation of the patient-physician relationship that is intrinsic to medicine. This patient-physician relationship is characterized by the goal of patient well-being and by the promise (literally, profession) of the physician to promote that goal.[8] Any physician involvement in efforts that might jeopardize the maximum benefit to any given patient would be thought to compromise the physician's core identity as patient advocate.

First, not to provide a possible benefit is to harm by omission. Second, it is to deny the unique vulnerability of the patient when it comes to standing up for himself or herself. The average patient possesses few resources that can help him or her identify and rectify the omissions of his or her physician. It seems a particularly pointed corruption of the physician's promise if he or she deepens the patient's vulnerability by way of hidden omissions. Failure to offer treatments of possible benefit would thus seem to erode the trust essential to the patient-physician relationship. We do not expect our physicians to put other concerns before our own well-being.

Additionally, negative gatekeeping could also violate truth telling and the open exchange of information. It can be argued that patients do not fully understand the incentive structures—like those of diagnosis-related groups (DRGs) and health maintenance organizations (HMOs), for example—that may limit tests or treatments of marginal benefit, and if they did know, the trust relationship with their physicians might be eroded. Their involuntary ignorance could also be construed as a violation of their autonomy. Patient autonomy could be considered to be violated as well if patients are not given the opportunity to accept or reject interventions of even marginal benefit.

Attention to the welfare of the individual patient as described above is at the very heart of medicine as a profession. Except for the most skeptical of accounts, a definition of professions seems always to include an account of the interplay of autonomy, responsibility, and service. Unlike other occupations, there is the assumption that professionals are not only, and perhaps not primarily, self-interested. Their activity is necessarily directed toward the benefit of others. Professions are understood according to this service component, and an argument against the involvement of physicians in cost containment is often based on the claim that considerations of cost are unprofessional. One commentator goes so far as to argue that asking physicians to be cost conscious would be asking them to "[r]emove the Hippocratic Oath from the waiting room walls and replace it with a sign that reads, "Warning all ye who enter here. I will generally work for your rights and welfare, but if benefits to you are marginal and costs are great, I will abandon you in order to protect society' " (p.14).[5]

In order for this sort of argument based on the concept of profession to succeed against gatekeeping, one would have to show that *only* the interests of particular patients, taken one at a time, are morally relevant. Yet practically speaking, physicians do speak of a duty to their practice, including the *group* of patients for whom they care. It is unclear why an understanding of profession as service would limit those served to those immediately seen. Profession, as described, includes a notion of expanded, not limited, sympathies. In fact, it can be argued that the concept of profession *requires* the consideration of justice as a necessary part of professional function.

First, denying patients access to services of marginal benefit does not obviate the possibility of the medical profession's promoting health, one of its primary objectives. If marginal care that is foregone enables other care of greater efficacy to be offered, the general goal of increased health is, in fact, promoted. Additionally, if we regard service as an essential component of professional duty, then service to all in need through the just allocation of resources seems to be a requirement for the fulfillment of professional function.

The argument seems to turn on what is meant by advocacy. In a more traditional framework, advocacy refers only to the welfare of the individual patient. Even if one accepts the claim that some party must assure the just allocation of health care, the physician could still act as an advocate for a particular patient against the vagaries of a social bureaucracy. In this scenario, physicians as individual patient advocates could provide a kind of system of checks and balances.

Yet advocacy might be better understood in less individualistic terms. Even granting that physicians have an obligation to benefit patients and protect them from impersonal bureaucracies and misguided policies, this might be more effectively accomplished if physicians have shared responsibility for cost containment on both the individual and the societal level. Absolute refusal to consider efficiency and cost could be viewed as being hostile to social concerns or as promoting the physician's self-interest. Exemption from considerations of cost and allocation might thereby compromise the physician's ability to advocate effectively on behalf of patients, whether his or her own, or all patients.

Norman Daniels identifies five key features of advocacy that do not necessarily conflict with the just allocation of health care or the physician's involvement in cost containment. If physicians are to be pure or ideal advocates for their patients, they should be (1) competent and up to the professional standards of care, (2) respectful of patient autonomy, (3) respectful of other patient rights—for example, confidentiality, (4) free from consideration of the physician's interests, and (5) uninfluenced by judgments about the patient's worth.[9] Physicians, in this view, may ethically consider costs as long as they have no personal economic interests in doing so, and as long as they do not judge whether a patient is worthy of particular treatment or not.

What is necessary is that physicians make their decisions within a system where resources are allocated fairly, where benefits foregone in one instance can be used to the greater benefit of others. These types of judgments about the just distribution of health care resources must be social and public ones. When a physician acts within such a system, he or she is abiding by a just social decision, not an idiosyncratic determination that it is not worth the resources to treat a particular patient in a particular way.[8]

Rethinking Patient Autonomy

The values and preferences of the particular patient are central to the traditional moral framework in medicine, and also central to a concept of advocacy. Negative physician gatekeeping could risk violating this important principle. How can the goals of just distribution of resources and respect for patient autonomy be reconciled?

One way to reconcile the two goals is by an expanded moral framework for medical decision making that emphasizes patient responsibility rather than autonomy. In an expanded framework that includes justice, it is not any choice that is valued, but the responsible choice. A responsible patient would be one concerned about the impact of his or her choice on others. In this sense, patient preference would not be solely self-regarding. We would thus alter our thinking about autonomy and patient preference sufficiently to allow room for some consideration of cost.

Understood in this way, respect for autonomy would require more discussion and openness concerning cost than now occurs. Currently, there are multiple barriers to the exchange of information about cost, including lack of information on the part of physicians and reluctance on their part to talk with patients about money. If one considers the individual's health to be of ultimate value, as many physicians do, then discussions of cost could indeed be considered irrelevent.

But there is increasing evidence that patients themselves are concerned about cost.[9] The difficulty is in translating a general concern into the needs of particular patients. As has been observed, the American public is somewhat schizophrenic when it comes to health care costs.[10] A majority want to control costs, and yet few want to change the status quo when it comes to individual health care decisions. There is no problem for patients who want to control costs and wish to consider them in their personal choices. But what about patients who also want costs to decrease, but who, when it comes to themselves, want everything done?

In more formal analysis, this is known as the problem of the "free rider." As indicated earlier, controlling the cost of health care is in everyone's interest. Yet at the same time it is always in any particular individual's interest to receive maximum service while everyone else does not. That way the individual receives the benefit of reduced expenditures and also still receives the benefit of the service. He or she has a free ride: obtaining the benefit without paying the full price. Ought we to require physicians to be advocates for free riders?

In order to take the position that they should be such advocates, one would have to argue that the principle of autonomy is far more important than other principles such as beneficence, in the form of benefits to be derived from reduced expenditures, and justice, in the form of the fair allocation of resources. Autonomy, though a central value, is not usually regarded as having such overriding importance. One of the accepted limits to personal freedom of choice is the harm that comes to others. It can be argued that total freedom to choose what to spend harms others in the form of increased expenditures and reduced availability.

Consent to a System of Cost Containment

Some kind of consent would seem necessary for cost-containment efforts in order to satisfy the physician's obligation to respect autonomy. But how is this to be implemented? Must a patient be informed of every possible procedure and benefit and be left to determine what benefits to forego on the basis of cost? Once the patient is advised of costs, should his or her preference determine whether a "marginal" service is provided?

Since truth telling is such an essential component of both autonomy and the patient-physician relationship, thorough disclosure of the reasons for physicians' recommendations would seem to be required. One of the major concerns raised about the British system of allocating certain forms of care is the perceived deception of patients by physicians and also of physicians by themselves. H. J. Aaron and W. B. Schwartz in *The Painful Prescription* describe how patients are not told about options that are deemed too costly, and should patients ask about them, they are told these options are not medically indicated.[11] The patient is led to believe that the decision is made on the basis of medical best interests rather than on cost-worthiness. The physician himself or herself often comes to believe that the decision rests on medical rather than economic grounds. In part because individual choice is secondary to the National Health Service's obligation to control expenditures through resource allocation, attention to informed consent is minimal in the British system.[12]

Yet Aaron and Schwartz also describe how British citizens are for the most part very pleased with their system.[11] Is this satisfaction based on ignorance of the true nature and extent of the rationing? Or does it represent implicit consent to the system that has developed? Insofar as the system is developed and maintained by a representative government, some kind of acceptance can be assumed when there is not widespread revolt against the system, or when it is not a central issue in elections.

In the United States, the same kind of political consent would seem possible regarding government programs. The question is more complicated here because of the decentralized nature of a health care system that includes both private and public providers and payment mechanisms. Presumably, though, some level of acceptance of cost-containment efforts on the part of private providers could be assumed if the consumer did not go elsewhere. But there are multiple problems with a concept of public consent that require more careful analysis.

A major limitation of this concept of consent through a political process or through purchase power is that patients/citizens/consumers may not be well informed and may acquiesce out of ignorance rather than out of reasoned agreement. The danger of simple acquiescence is especially true in health care which is complex and very important to the lives of people often made particularly vulnerable through illness.

For many medical procedures, information about effectiveness is in the form of statistical statements which may be difficult for patients to comprehend. Even more troublesome, much of medical decision making must confront vast areas of uncertainty. Outcomes may be unpredictably altered by biological phenomena that are little understood, human variability, and even subtle differences in skill and use of procedures. Since many interventions require a complex combination of activities, it is very difficult for patients to judge quality except in a very global way. For the patient who is already anxious and feeling ill, such barriers to understanding may be all but insurmountable. Our belief in informed consent requires that patients be informed of medical risks and benefits in these situations and be permitted to choose accordingly. The physician bears responsibility for guiding patients through the thicket of ambiguity. Asking patients to act as true consumers, weighing risks, benefits, *and* costs, may be asking the impossible, especially when they are already compromised by illness. It is because people are neither accustomed to acting nor truly able to act as independent consumers that it is risky to regard health care as just another commodity under market control.[12]

Another impediment to the consumer-provider model in health care arises with respect to freedom of choice. Even if patients could unequivocally identify their needs, which is doubtful, they often face severely limited choices. A person who falls ill in one community may not be medically stable enough to go elsewhere, irrespective of his or her preferences. Patients may be unable, then, to take their business to another provider of care when they are dissatisfied. Once again, acquiescence, not consent, may occur.

Yet another danger is that societal consent may be interpreted too broadly and abstractly. A general interest on the part of the public in controlling health care costs cannot be interpreted as a consent not to receive dialysis, for example. Decisions regarding standards for weighing what care is to be provided and what is to be foregone must be made in an open fashion. The general public must be aware of the nature and extent of cost-containment measures and have recourse to change.

But if there is a process whereby information is provided, and if there is sufficient opportunity for response, so that patients and physicians may change cost-containment measures that are thought too detrimental, then public consent can have some weight. Physicians, in this setting, are not required to be free rider advocates. The principle of autonomy is balanced with beneficence and justice, and individual advocacy is balanced with individual responsibility to others in the community. The only way theoretically to bridge the gap between the individual patient and all patients, and still maintain the role of patient advocate, is to argue that patients themselves are already responsible to each other and to all. Patients are not isolated from the requirements of justice, and, therefore, physicians are not required to act as though they were.

AN ARGUMENT SUPPORTING PHYSICIAN GATEKEEPING

Thus far, we have described a principle of justice as fairness that would preclude some individuals from having unlimited access to health care while others had virtually none. Cost containment is one of several approaches to assuring sufficient resources to meet a society's health care needs. We have noted that there appears to be a general sentiment supporting efforts to control costs, but that the nature and scope of such activities will require open and informed public debate. Finally, we have argued that the right of individuals to direct their own care is legitimately constrained by a responsibility, as members of a community, to uphold the requirements of justice in health care. Physicians, like their patients, have obligations of justice, as well as beneficence and respect for autonomy. Their role is not that of advocate for the unrestrained marginal choice or the free rider, but of advocate for the patient in the context of shared responsibility to assure just allocation of resources. Gatekeeping, then, is part of that shared responsibility.

If society takes seriously its obligation to allocate health care resources justly, then the role of physicians will be critical. A just allocation cannot be accomplished without physician involvement. Physician expertise includes effectiveness and efficiency in the use of tests and treatments. Guiding the patient away from interventions of marginal benefit and significant cost and educating patients to understand and cope with the uncertainties inherent in medical care are important tasks that physicians are best able to accomplish. Physicians will not only further the goals of justice, but also enhance the position of patients as well-informed participants in individual and societal choices. Explicit discussions of the reasons for deciding against one option and for another will permit physician and patient to maximize benefit and minimize harm for both the individual and the community.

In fact, one might argue that physicians who continue to act "as if" no constraints existed will only perpetuate current injustices. To the extent that some patients are reinforced either in the illusion that no constraints exist or in more cynical free-ridership, misallocation of resources is likely to continue. In all likelihood, it will be the most vulnerable members of society, those lacking the political, economic, or physical resources to protest, who will remain underserved, while others continue to receive unlimited care. Responsible physician-gatekeepers can serve as de facto advocates for this group of individuals in particular.

Additionally, the concept of the physician as one who can only swing the gate open reflects a diminished notion of professional autonomy. It presumes that the physician only acts as a procurer between the patient and a desired resource. In fact, physicians have always retained the legitimate obligation to say "no" as well as "yes." Beneficence requires that physicians argue against or even refuse to participate in care that is only harmful or clearly worthless.

Physician autonomy can also be compromised if physicians are completely excluded from allocation decisions. Having others make allocation decisions would reduce the occasions when physicians themselves must say "no" to patients, but at the high price of also limiting the physician's opportunity to say "yes." If others make all decisions, they will be the ones practicing medicine, and without a license.[13]

If, as we have said, benefit to others is contingent on care in the use of resources, and if harm will result if such care is not taken, then physicians must be able to say "no" to noncost-worthy interventions in the discharge of their professional role. The constraint here is similar to that which applies in the case of a "pure" medical judgment. Cost-worthiness must be based on the medical condition of the patient (which physicians must be free to judge) and on the conclusions of social debates, not on the idiosyncratic judgments of individual physicians with regard to the value or worth of any particular patient.

One final caveat remains. Societal decisions to allocate health care resources fairly legitimize gatekeeping to the extent that the gatekeeping furthers the availability of health care generally. It would seem an abuse of the responsible physician and patient alike if the resources they gave up did not contribute to this overall goal. Cost containment that does not contribute to the correction of misallocation loses its moral justification. It is essential, therefore, that every effort be expended to assure that the system overall reflects the concern for justice that motivates the physician-gatekeeper and his or her patient.

Expenditures for health care cannot continue their upward spiral forever without endangering other goods society considers essential. Justice as fairness requires that whatever is spent on health care provides access to a basic level of care for everyone. Ensuring a just distribution of health care resources is the responsibility of each member of society and is intrinsic to every medical decision. Physician reimbursement schemes that provide incentives to lower costs and provide services more efficiently are justified insofar as they promote the just allocation of health care resources generally.

NOTES

1. J. M. Eisenberg, *Doctors' Decisions and the Cost of Medical Care* (Ann Arbor, Mich.: Health Administration Press Perspectives, 1986), p. 3.

2. A. Enthoven and R. Kronick, "A Consumer-Choice Health Plan for the 1990's, Universal Health Insurance in a System Designed to Promote Quality and Economy (First of Two Parts)," *New England Journal of Medicine* 320 (1989): 29.

3. President's Commission for the Study of Ethical Problems in Medicine and Biomedical and Behavioral Research, *Securing Access to Health Care: The Ethical Implications of Differences in the Availability of Health Services* (Washington, D.C.: U.S. Government Printing Office, 1983).

4. R. Veatch, *A Theory of Medical Ethics* (New York: Basic Books, 1981).

5. R. Veatch, "The HMO Physician's Duty to Cut Costs," *Hastings Center Report* 15:4 (August 1985): 13–14.

6. R. Veatch, "DRG's and the Ethical Reallocation of Resources," *Hastings Center Report* 16:3 (June 1986): 32–40.

7. R. Veatch, *The Foundations of Justice* (London: Oxford University Press, 1986), pp. 181–83.

8. E. Pellegrino and D. Thomasma, *A Philosophical Basis of Medical Practice: Toward a Philosophy and Ethic of the Healing Professions* (London: Oxford University Press, 1981), pp. 209–10.

9. N. Daniels, "The Ideal Advocate and Limited Resources," *Theoretical Medicine* 8:1 (1987): 69–80.

10. R. Blenden and D. Altman, "Public Attitudes About Health Care Costs: A Lesson in National Schizophrenia," *New England Journal of Medicine* 31:9 (1984): 613–16.

11. H. J. Aaron and W. B. Schwartz, *The Painful Prescription: Rationing Health Care* (Washington, D.C.: Brookings Institution, 1984), pp. 100–102.

12. R. Schwartz and A. Grubb, "Why Britain Can't Afford Informed Consent," *Hastings Center Report* 15:4 (August 1985): 19–25.

13. E. H. Morreim, "Clinicians or Committees—Who Should Cut Costs?" *Hastings Center Report* 17:2 (1987): 45.

3

Assessing and Paying for Quality

Molla Donaldson

"Paying the doctor" is no longer just a matter of contracting or paying for physician services. It is rapidly becoming an issue of "paying for quality." Purchasers, particularly large, third-party purchasers, would like to move beyond the standard utilization review approaches of cost containment, such as claims review and precertification.[1, 2] They are trying to develop strategies to identify levels of quality and translate such information into purchasing decisions.[3] This effort is well underway and will undoubtedly be occurring with increasing intensity. How well informed or misguided such attempts may be is the subject of this chapter.

PAYING FOR QUALITY

There is an adage that "you get what you pay for." Until recently, however, both individual and third-party payers have been paying for whatever they got, with the price largely unknown beforehand and the quality (what you get) unknown either before or after care was rendered. With the extraordinary rise in health care costs, particularly in costs for physicians' services, payers of all kinds, both corporate and public, have been asking with increasing frequency and frustration, "What are we getting?" "Is the health of our employees, retirees, or poor citizens really better now, just the same, or worse than it was when we were paying a fraction of these charges?"

More ominously the question is sometimes phrased, "How much can we cut down on what we pay before our beneficiaries experience adverse health outcomes?" No one has asked this question seriously before, but now not only is it being asked, but also tentative answers are being attempted.

Hospital care is currently the primary target of such questions because costs are so great, outcomes so dramatic, and data relatively more plentiful. The huge Medicare data base for Part A claims, which largely represent hospital charges, is being supplemented by hospital data from many other payers.[4] These data are supplied by hospitals to state health care cost-containment commissions and state hospital associations. The data can be aggregated and analyzed to produce medical and surgical discharge rates and outcome indicators such as hospital-specific rates of mortality, surgical complications, nosocomial (hospital-acquired) infections, and readmissions. Many observers are hopeful these data will allow quality comparisons that will inform purchasing decisions.

The concern about hospital costs and resulting cost-containment efforts by third-party payers, as well as the implementation of the Medicare prospective payments system, has resulted in a rapid shift in the location of care for numerous diagnostic and surgical procedures. Procedures such as lens extraction, arthroscopy (using a small beam of light to view a joint), and hernia repair were until very recently performed in the hospital. Many procedures are now performed in ambulatory surgical centers, outpatient clinics, and private offices. This shift has moved services out of the Part A claims base and the attendant scrutiny and into Medicare Part B claims, the data system for physician services.

Despite the shift in location, the question "What are we getting?" remains, and it will undoubtedly lead to more determined calls for data about the benefit of the care. In other words, questions about quality and appropriateness will be applied increasingly not only to the institutional setting such as the hospital, but also to the doctor's office; in fact, legislation has called for Medicare review of ambulatory physicians' services to begin in 1990.

Concerns about costs have been accompanied by greater interest in selective contracting and by interest in managed care and preferred provider organizations. In these systems the performance of physicians, in relation both to the charges they generate and to the quality of care they provide, can (at least in theory) be monitored, analyzed by individual, and used to determine physician payments.[5]

Employers and business coalitions throughout the country are developing and implementing plans for value purchasing, an idea advanced by Walter McClure, embraced by numerous corporations as a stated goal in health care purchasing, and a driving force in the acquisition and distribution of quality data. The effort is based on the assumption that distribution of data will result in competition based not only on cost and benefit levels, but also on quality.[6, 7, 8, 9, 10] The intent of these programs is to force out poor high-cost providers unless they improve enough to become more competitive.

But what is quality, and what methods are available to identify and accurately link it to payment? Are there reliable and valid tools of assessment available to purchasers?

CRITERIA FOR JUDGING QUALITY

Over twenty years ago Avedis Donabedian[11] described health care as including three measurable components: structure, process, and outcome.

Structure refers to the capacity for high-quality care encompassed by such attributes as staffing, facilities, and policies. Process refers to those technical maneuvers such as history taking, diagnostic testing, and therapeutic interventions initiated by practitioners as well as the interpersonal process sometimes referred to as the "art of care." This includes listening, answering questions, and informing patients so that they may share in decision making and in their own self-care. Outcome refers both to the short-term consequences of particular treatment, such as control of blood pressure, and to long-term patient health status, including death. Outcomes are the most appealing to purchasers as a measure of quality because they represent what is most sought (or avoided) in health care.

All three characteristics—structure, process, and outcome—have been extraordinarily useful in formulating and conducting research studies on quality. Controversy has been considerable, however, concerning the relationship between structure, process, and outcome. Can poor structure or process be linked in practice to poor outcome? Conversely, and more problematic, is it possible to link good outcome with prior good structure or process?[12, 13] The answers to such questions become crucial when purchasers intend to use good or poor outcomes to make generalizations about the quality of providers.

QUALITY OF CARE: AN INDUSTRIAL ANALOGY

When we consider health care in comparison to industrial production, we do not find it hard to understand why a definitive linkage among structure, process, and outcome is so difficult. Consider "high-quality" industrial production. The environment (e.g., temperature, air quality) is kept constant, inputs are as uniform as possible, and the process is carefully specified. The workers assigned to a given task have comparable training and are consistent in behavior, and the output can be examined, rejected, or reworked. The cybernetic cycle in which a problem in output leads to modification in input or process is well established. Some industrial settings might be less fastidious, but it is improbable that a high-quality product (something that conforms to specifications and is suitable for the use intended) will result without the foregoing steps.

Now consider the health care production "hopper."

Environment

Surrounding the hopper is the health care environment—reimbursement, competition, malpractice, education, worker and facility availability, and regulation. Elements of the environment change continuously, faster than research and demonstration projects can assess their influence. Furthermore, the environment varies dramatically from one area to the next. For example, states have varying regulations concerning health care practices; even within states and regions, conditions vary greatly in such domains as the supply of health care professionals and facilities, attitudes toward capitated arrangements, the influence of medical associations, and business-labor relations.

Structure

Inside the structural part of the hopper is a slurry of policies and practices pertaining to facility design, equipment, personnel, credentials, communication, and information systems.

Two input streams flow into the hopper. The patient stream reflects various patient characteristics. These may be discrete (e.g., gender, symptoms, Activities of Daily Living), elongate (e.g., age, stage of disease), of different sizes (e.g., comorbidities and past medical history), or fuzzy (e.g., health beliefs, cultural attitude, social support, genetic predisposition).

The practitioner stream includes varying levels of training (e.g., technician, aide, nurse, primary care physician, subspecialty, critical care), experience, skill, and all the personal characteristics of the patient stream.

Process

The combined streams move in a more or less linear fashion into the "process" part of the hopper. Here are clouds of diagnostic tests, procedures, and therapeutic alternatives (e.g., no or delayed intervention, surgery, or drugs, alone and in all possible combinations).

Outcome

The most salient fact about the outcome portion of the hopper is that the product is unseen. Typically, outcomes are unmeasured, unrecorded, and unknown. Infrequent and isolated events are retrieved and recorded as elements of "claims data" or "reportable events"—death, readmission to hospital, nosocomial infections, complications, disenrollment—but these may not be the outcomes of greatest interest to patients. One analyst likened the use of mortality data as the only measure of the outcome of care to a scale with only zero or one hundred on it.

Although data in claims may be accurate for those elements of care on which payment depends, other elements may or may not be recorded and, if recorded, may or may not be accurate.[14, 15, 16, 17] Outcomes of care, such as complications, that may be used to criticize a practitioner's performance, especially by those who are not professional peers, are unlikely to be recorded with great precision. This realization has led researchers to seek "nonintrusive" outcomes—that is, outcomes that do not depend on voluntary recording by health professionals.

Another form of recording bias was documented by Stephen Jencks[18] and his colleagues.[19] They demonstrated that covariants (such as other conditions present at the time of a hospital admission that may contribute to a patient death) are less likely to have been recorded for patients with poor outcomes than for those with good outcomes.

MEASURING QUALITY AND LINKING STRUCTURE, PROCESS, AND OUTCOME MEASURES

Environmental, patient, and provider characteristics affect choices among sometimes hundreds of diagnostic and therapeutic options, few of which have been rigorously linked to outcomes that control for more than a few variables. It should be evident why linking the rare identified outcome with a particular structural feature, diagnostic decision, or therapeutic choice would be extraordinarily difficult. This is *not* a connect-the-dots endeavor. Yet the thrust of most efforts at rating and comparing providers relies on outcome measurement.

Paul Ellwood has written about a technology of outcomes management as a way of appropriately restoring competition based on quality to the medical market.[19] Outcome data must, however, be seen as a first screen to indicate what to review more carefully. Mortality rates, for instance, have been touted as a good place to begin to look at the quality of hospitals. In theory, if observed deaths exceed the expected number of deaths in a given facility, it is tempting for purchasers to conclude that the quality of care is low in that facility and that the "excess" deaths were preventable. But mortality rates by themselves provide no information about quality. Even after ensuring that an acceptable measurement of mortality is used (e.g., thirty days after hospital admission), and that an adequate number of cases over a period of time have been reviewed to provide statistical significance, one would need to know what is to be considered a "preventable" death.

One hospital medical director described how his hospital had been bannered in the newspapers for having the worst care in the community because four "preventable" deaths had been attributed to it. Examination by the hospital medical staff showed that all four had been cases of acute myocardial infarction. One case had been pronounced dead on arrival at the hospital. One had been resuscitated multiple times in the emergency room and had died subsequently in the intensive care unit. The hospital conceded this might have been preventable. The remaining two cases had been resuscitated, stabilized, discharged appropriately, and later admitted to other hospitals where they had died. Both of these deaths were attributed to the first hospital. The mortality rate did not, by itself, illuminate the pattern of quality of care in that community. Perhaps there were quality problems, but they might have been associated more with emergency medical services provided by the city or with care received in other hospitals than with the care rendered in the cited hospital.

Efforts to refine mortality rates are well underway, in particular, by the use of risk adjustment to account for patients of differing levels of severity of illness, ages, and sexes at the time of their admission.[20, 21, 22, 23, 24, 25, 26, 27] Such risk-adjusted mortality by facility might then be compared by surgical procedure or medical reason for admission to that of other facilities and lead to case review.

Valuable information about patient care can be gained from review of the records of patients having some adverse outcome. An internal quality assurance program, for instance, might find many areas needing improvement while reviewing any given case. This is because, in general, any area of medical care that is scrutinized will quickly yield numerous problem areas that might be followed up with action or further sampling and review. How is quality determined by case review?

Two elements are required for a valid determination of the quality of the process of care. First, there must be valid and reliable information about the efficacy of a given element of care (the probability of benefit to individuals in a defined population from a medical technology* applied for a given medical problem under ideal conditions of use[28]) and its effectiveness (the probability of benefit when medical technology is applied under ordinary conditions by the average practitioner for the typical patient)[29] such that a practice standard can be set. Second, there must be a measure of performance using that standard. As David Eddy[30] has eloquently shown, demonstrations of the first kind are rare. Unlike drugs that must be shown to be efficacious before they are introduced on the market, diagnostic and therapeutic procedures have no such requirement. Resources have been scarce for controlled clinical trials, and even when such trials are performed, only a few of the pertinent variables can be controlled. Those who would measure quality generally have acted without such solid information about efficacy and effectiveness and have based criteria on clinical consensus about accepted or best practices. These vary widely in methods of development

---

*The term *technology* might be used very broadly in quality assessment to include not only such obvious technologies as diagnostic procedures, but also, for instance, managed care arrangements, surgical procedures, drug intervention, or case management.

from "tuna fish" guidelines for a review of care (developed over lunch by several busy clinicians) to the convening of expert panels to use their clinical experience to set criteria on the assumption that a correct process will, in some way, be related to a favorable outcome. For the second requirement, quality assessment based on well-validated elements of care, numerous methods have been developed, often involving record review using a formalized auditing process and sometimes several layers of review with successively more specialized clinical expertise. Other methods involve patient interview and claims analysis. Patient preferences can be elicited and combined with therapeutic options in these guidelines. During data analysis, multivariate statistical techniques can then sort, combine, and clarify the relative contributions of patient and provider characteristics and behavior to a given outcome of care.

The current state of quality assessment is such that the *process* of care by settings, practitioners, or groups of patients can be assessed according to predetermined standards for those areas in which efficacy and effectiveness are known or exist by consensus. Measures include such aspects of care as technical competence, accessibility, acceptability, satisfaction, coordination and continuity, humanistic behavior, and patient education.

For most areas, the science of assessment is still rudimentary, rarely validated, and highly variable depending on the setting and the patient population. Such efforts are advanced, however, in comparison to our ability to move from "poor" or "adverse" outcomes, such as death or readmission, to a defective process element. Current science will not allow a poor outcome to be considered de facto evidence of poor quality.

An external purchaser of care who wants to use outcome data for quality ratings, and thus decide whether to purchase care, might do so by following either of two strategies: (1) The purchaser might decide it does not care what kind of processes led to the events. That the provider was an outlier after risk adjustments have been made to the data is sufficient to disqualify it (or him or her) from participation (at the risk of excluding good providers). (2) The purchaser might combine this information with other process data about the provider in the hope of building a composite and consistent profile of care. This is would be a very difficult course to choose because consistency requires that multiple measures lead to the same relative rating and that scores over time are consistent. If either the scores over time or the results of multiple measures are inconsistent, the purchaser must determine which measures or time periods are most important. It is not hard, for instance, to imagine satisfied patients whose providers have no specialty board certification; care that ranked low on certain measures, but has been improving over time; very difficult access—for example, waiting times, hours of operation, geographic isolation—but wonderful interpersonal skills; extraordinary success with very difficult cases, but perhaps overzealous intervention. It would be up to the purchaser to construct a composite rating that would reflect the providers' priorities (though not necessarily those of the beneficiaries).

Currently, no mechanism describes how to weigh and summarize quality of care "scores" for a given provider or organization such that one score can meaningfully be compared with any other. Any such system would be purely idiosyncratic, based on the personal bias of the score constructor and, incidentally, extraordinarily expensive to do with any level of thoroughness. The cost of such evaluation, would, of course, have to be built into the cost of care.

CURRENT EFFORTS UNDER WAY

What is the current state of the art? Where are purchasers now in this difficult attempt to devise a valid way of "paying for quality?" How can a purchaser know who the high- or low-quality providers are and incorporate this into prospective purchasing decisions? In brief, the process has just begun.

Purchasers have begun to explore how to apply the findings of a series of studies done by researchers at the RAND Corporation. The studies used an exhaustive process including expert consensus panels to identify clearly appropriate or inappropriate circumstances for such procedures as carotid endarterectomy, endoscopy, and coronary angiography.[31, 32] Appropriate use of such diagnostic procedures could be considered a marker of quality that could then be linked to prospective purchasing and to both prospective and retrospective payment denial.

William Roper, the administrator of the Health Care Financing Administration (HCFA) at the U.S. Department of Health and Human Services in the Reagan administration, oversaw what has become an almost routine release of hospital-specific mortality data for the stated purpose of helping patients choose their hospitals. But there has also been recognition that quality assessment cannot proceed very far without a more scientific base of effective practice. Before leaving the HCFA, Roper undertook a new effectiveness initiative.[33] Under contract with the HCFA, the Institute of Medicine has conducted a series of effectiveness initiative workshops that sought to identify conditions and patient management steps where effectiveness can be established.[34] Since the HCFA manages the Medicare program, its reimbursement decisions are likely to drive decision making throughout the health care delivery system. Health policy experts and the Physician Payment Review Commission (PPRC) have called for federal support for effectiveness research and practice guidelines.[35, 36]

Purchasers have concentrated on the areas of mandating case-mix adjustments, contracting selectively for specialized services, developing preferred provider organizations (PPOs), mandating and developing uniform clinical data sets,[9, 37] and experimenting with such communitywide approaches as the Rochester Area Hospital Experimental Payments Program and the Pennsylvania Buy Right Council in Pittsburgh. In the Rochester experiment the hospitals in the community have agreed to disburse a small percentage of pooled revenues based on quality performance. In the Pennsylvania program Walter McClure has espoused the "buy right" strategy in which purchasers act in concert within a community and require certain uniform data from providers in order to make contracting decisions based on performance as well as price. A central piece in this strategy is the use of proprietary case-mix-adjusting software.

A number of states, notably Colorado, Iowa, and Pennsylvania, have demonstrated their interest in the use of cost and quality data. As a result of state legislation, all Pennsylvania hospitals have been required to install the MedisGroups severity software to provide the state with required case-mix-adjusted data on costs and outcomes. The Pennsylvania Health Care Cost Containment Commission has published a report on costs per case and the morbidity and mortality rates of each Pennsylvania hospital. The Cost Containment Commission's Data Council intends that the data it provides will help business and labor purchasers make cost- and quality-informed choices in purchasing care for their beneficiaries. The Honeywell Corporation is seeking physician data from Blue Cross–Blue Shield of Minnesota. Honeywell plans to use the claims data to profile the high- and low-cost physicians, to identify those providing better or worse care, and to use these data to steer its employees toward (or away from) individual practitioners by the use of differentials in cost sharing. The Washington, New York, and Midwest Business Groups on Health, as well as the Seattle Health Care Coalition, have been leaders in exploring the uses of data to enable corporations to develop strategies for value purchasing. A grant from the Hartford Foundation enabled the Midwest Business Group on Health to evaluate current efforts and produce a series of publications on value-managed health care purchasing.[9]

At a more advanced level, value purchasing might involve comparing performance on the basis of agreed-on measures of quality—that is, on measures chosen by the payer to represent those aspects of care thought to represent quality. These might be structural features, such as availability of after-hours care or the number of board-certified specialty physicians; process features, such as waiting times, compliance with cancer screening tests, or the appropriate use of surgical procedures; or outcome measures, such as a hospital infection rate or the disenrollment rate in a managed care plan. The Orange County Health Planning Council has developed such a tool to compare hospital performance.[38] The congressional Office of Technology Assessment (OTA) has developed an extensive list of possible measures of quality for use by consumers.[39] Although such methods would be equally applicable for the use of group purchasers, the study was not sanguine about the strength of the indicators it reviewed.

Health care organizations have themselves sought to reward high quality with monetary incentives. For instance, U.S. Healthcare, a New Jersey–based independent practice association, builds into its physician bonus program a formula that includes rates of patient transfers, patient satisfaction ratings, and the results of chart review.

It may become possible not only to measure outcomes of interest, but also to relate them to the process and structure of care such that purchasers can identify those providers that are offering especially good or especially poor care. However, there remains a major difficulty. All the above examples of efforts to define and pay for quality (or to avoid paying for poor quality) have the same pitfall. Assuming current efforts are refined so that we can accurately isolate those variations in patient outcomes attributable to medical care received, this would provide a guide to "quality" only under very specific circumstances: for given medical conditions, and at a single point of time—an indication of the *incidence* of quality. For selective contracting, a term that implies an ongoing relationship, one would prefer measures of the *prevalence* of quality for a given provider or organization and of the *trajectory* of quality. Does the organization have an internal program that actively seeks out and attempts to resolve problems? Is the practitioner continuing to develop his skills? Does he or she voluntarily engage in a peer review process? Ideally, a measure of quality should indicate the practitioner's or organization's capacity for and commitment to improvement and its changing performance over time; ideally, the purchaser should use its payment mechanisms to encourage improvement, not simply to penalize poor outcomes or decisions that occurred in the past. Some medical analysts leading internal quality assessment programs, notably Donald Berwick at the Harvard Community Health Plan and Paul Batalden at the Hospital Corporation of America, have encouraged group health care purchasers to think about long-term relationships with provider groups, to focus on quality improvement rather than on quality assessment, and to emulate the models of continuous improvement. Based on the work of W. Edwards Deming, Joseph J. Juran, and Philip B. Crosby, the continuous improvement model has been applied with reported success first in Japanese and subsequently in segments of American industry during the 1980s.

Entering a contract relationship may require only that performance at a given time be above a stated threshold. Once this decision is made and an ongoing relationship is sought, however, the purchaser needs to adopt a different strategy. At this point the quality assurance function (correcting problems and improving quality generally), in addition to quality assessment, probably becomes more important; that is, the determination with which an organization seeks and resolves problems may become a better test of its quality than minimal performance ratings. Decisions about terminating a contracting relationship may require elements of both.

CONCLUSION

The search will continue for simple outcome measures, preferably captured in large administrative data bases. Despite warnings, they may be taken at face value as quality measures.

Now the yield of "true" quality problems from all screens is uncertain and to date represents only a very small fraction of cases that are reviewed. As better measures are developed, it may be possible to increase the sensitivity and specificity of such outcome measures as quality screens.

In the meantime, composite process measures, probably in combination with outcome measures, may be the most promising strategy for "paying for quality." This approach will require far more research to determine which measures are most valid, will be very expensive to implement, and should be linked to incentives for improvement.

NOTES

The views expressed here are the author's and do not represent those of the Institute of Medicine and the National Academy of Science.

1. C. Inlander, "Consumers' Group Asks: Whose Life Is It Anyway?" *Business and Health* (September 1984): 28–30.

2. D. Awine, "Buyers Are Smarter, Looking for Quality," *Modern Healthcare* (1987): 32.

3. A. Enthoven and R. Kronick, "Competition 101: Managing Demand to Get Quality Care," *Business and Health* (March 1988): 38–40.

4. P. Caper, "The Epidemiologic Surveillance of Medical Care," *American Journal of Public Health* 77:6 (1987): 669–70.

5. R. H. Palmer, "The Challenges and Prospects for Quality Assessment and Assurance in Ambulatory Care," *Inquiry* 25:1 (1988): 119–31.

6. W. McClure, "Buying Right: The Consequences of Glut," *Business and Health* (September 1985): 43–46.

7. W. McClure, "Buying Right: How To Do It," *Business and Health* (October 1985): 41–44.

8. L. Wyszewianski, "Quality of Care: Past Achievements and Future Challenges," *Inquiry* 25:1 (1988): 13–22.

9. M. R. Chassin, J. Kosecoff, and R. Dubois, *Value-Managed Health Care Purchasing: An Employer's Guidebook Series* (Chicago: Midwest Business Group on Health, 1989).

10. P. E. Ellwood, "Banking on Quality," *HMO Practice* 2 (1988): 101–5.

11. A. Donabedian, "Evaluating the Quality of Medical Care," *Milbank Memorial Fund Quarterly* 44 (1966): 166–206.

12. A. Donabedian, *Explorations in Quality Assessment and Monitoring*, vol. 1, *The Definition of Quality and Approaches to Its Assessment* (Ann Arbor, Mich.: Health Administration Press, 1980).

13. K. N. Lohr, "Outcome Measurement: Concepts and Questions," *Inquiry* 25 (1988): 37–50.

14. Institute of Medicine, *Reliability of Hospital Discharge Abstracts*, IOM–77–01 (Washington, D.C.: National Academy Press, 1977).

15. Institute of Medicine, *Reliability of Hospital Discharge Records* IOM–77–05 (Washington, D.C.: National Academy Press, 1977).

16. Institute of Medicine, *Reliability of Hospital Discharge Records*, IOM–80–02 (Washington, D.C.: National Academy Press, 1980).

17. D. C. Hsia et al., "Accuracy of Diagnostic Coding for Medicare Patients under the Prospective Payment System," *New England Journal of Medicine* 318:6 (1988): 352–55.

18. S. F. Jencks, D. K. Williams, and T. L. Kay, "Assessing Hospital-Associated Deaths from Discharge Data: The Role of Length of Stay and Comorbidities," *Journal of the American Medical Association* 260 (1988): 2240–46.

19. P. M. Ellwood, "Outcomes Management: A Technology of Patient Experience," *New England Journal of Medicine* 318:23 (1988): 1549–56.

20. S. F. Jencks, "Case-Mix Measurement and Assessment Quality Hospital Care," *Health Care Finance Review* (annual supplement) (1987): 39–48.

21. J. Daley et al., "Predicting Hospital-Associated Mortality for Medicare Patients," *Journal of the American Medical Association* 260:24 (1988): 3617–24.

22. R. W. Dubois, R. H. Brook, and W. H. Rogers, "Adjusted Hospital Death Rates: A Potential Screen for Quality of Medical Care," *American Journal of Public Health* 77 (1987): 1162–66.

23. R. W. Dubois, J. H. Moxley, D. Draper, and R. H. Brook, "Hospital Inpatient Mortality: Is It a Predictor of Quality?" *New England Journal of Medicine* 317 (1987): 1674–80.

24. K. L. Kahn et al., "Interpreting Hospital Mortality Data: How Can We Proceed?" *Journal of the American Medical Association* 260 (1988): 3625–28.

25. S. F. Jencks, J. Dale, and D. Draper, "Interpreting Hospital Mortality Data: The Role of Clinical Risk Adjustment," *Journal of the American Medical Association* 260 (1988): 3611–16.

26. S. F. Greenfield, "Flaws in Mortality Data: The Hazards of Ignoring Comorbid Disease," *Journal of the American Medical Association* 260 (1988): 2253–55.

27. B. H. Ente and J. S. Lloyd, "Taking Stock of Mortality Data: A Joint Commission Conference," *Quarterly Review Bulletin* 15 (February 1989): 54–57.

28. U.S. Congress, Office of Technology Assessment, *Assessing the Efficacy and Safety of Medical Technologies*, OTA–H–75 (Washington, D.C.: Office of Technology Assessment, 1978), p. 16.

29. R. H. Brook and K. N. Lohr, "Efficacy, Effectiveness, Variations, and Quality: Boundary Crossing Research," *Medical Care* 23 (May 1985): 711.

30. D. M. Eddy and J. Billings, "The Quality of Medical Evidence: Implications for Quality of Care," *Health Affairs* 7:4 (1988): 19–32.

31. M. R. Chassin et al., "Does Inappropriate Use Explain Geographic Variations in the Use of Health Services? A Study of Three Procedures," *Journal of the American Medical Association* 259 (1987): 2533–37.

32. J. Kosecoff et al., "Obtaining Clinical Data on the Appropriateness of Medical

Care in Community Practice," *Journal of the American Medical Association* 258 (1987): 2538–42.

33. W. L. Roper et al., "Effectiveness in Health Care: An Initiative to Evaluate and Improve Medical Practice," *New England Journal of Medicine* 319:18 (1988): 1197–1202.

34. Institute of Medicine, *Report of a Study. Effectiveness Initiative: Setting Priorities for Clinical Conditions* (Washington, D.C.: National Academy Press, 1980).

35. Physician Payment Review Commission, *Annual Report to Congress* (Washington, D.C.: U.S. Government Printing Office, 1989).

36. A. S. Relman, "Assessment and Accountability: The Third Revolution in Medical Care," *New England Journal of Medicine* 319:18 (1988): 1220–22.

37. Colorado Health Data Commission, "The Application of a Uniform Clinical Data Set to the Assessment of Severity-Adjusted Care Outcomes for Hospital Inpatients Project Description" (Colorado Health Data Commission, July 1988, Typescript).

38. F. Bodendorf and F. G. Mackey, *A Hospital's IQ: Indicators of Quality* (Tustin, Calif.: Orange County Health Planning Council, 1985).

39. U.S. Congress, Office of Technology Assessment, *The Quality of Medical Care: Information for Consumers*, OTA–H–386 (Washington, D.C.: U.S. Government Printing Office, June 1988).

4

Physician Reimbursement: The Lessons of Economics

Mary Ann Baily

How should physicians be paid? The answer to the question depends on the end that is sought. In broad terms, most people would probably say they want the "right" amounts and quality levels of physician services produced and delivered to the "right" people, they want physicians to receive a "fair" reward for their efforts, and they prefer not to sacrifice any more than necessary of other goods and services to achieve this. In other words, the goal is a payment system that is both efficient and equitable.

THE MARKET MODEL

What can economics contribute to understanding this question? The basic model in economics is that of the *market*—the interaction of buyers and sellers that determines what is produced and how it is distributed. The key to the operation of a market is the *price*, which mediates between those offering a good and those seeking it. When the quantity demanded exceeds the quantity supplied, price rises, sellers offer more, and buyers want less; when the quantity supplied is in excess, price falls. In other words, prices and quantities adjust until what is bought equals what is sold, and, in economic jargon, the market is in equilibrium.

Economists spend much of their effort analyzing the factors that influence buyer and seller behavior and the resulting market equilibrium. In an economic system such as ours, in which most goods (including medical care) are allocated through a system of interconnected markets, this analysis is a powerful tool. It can be used to explain existing patterns of production and distribution and to predict what will happen when the factors that have determined them change, whether as a consequence of natural events (failure of the wheat crop in the Midwest) or of public policies (import quotas on Japanese cars).

The market model has more than descriptive value, however. Economists focus on markets not only because markets are *there*, but also because, to economists, they are *good*. It is useful to understand why economists value markets so highly, so that when market outcomes prove undesirable in practice, one can more easily understand what has gone wrong.

Economists like markets for their ability to allocate resources efficiently. In the economic theory of market behavior, when price harmonizes decisions to buy a good with offers to sell, it harmonizes the preferences of consumers with societal resources. On the demand side, consumers are assumed to make purchases to maximize the satisfaction they get from their budgets. This means that when buying something, consumers consider the extra satisfaction (the marginal utility) another unit of the good will give them, compare it to the price, and decide if it is worth it. On the supply side, the good's producers are assumed to maximize profits. They consider the additional cost of supplying another unit (the marginal cost) and compare it to the price.

In a system of well-functioning markets, the marginal resource cost represents the opportunity cost to society of another unit of the good—what must be given up elsewhere in the economy to have it. At market equilibrium, therefore, the benefit to consumers of having a little more of the good has automatically been brought into line with its cost.

A major advantage of this process is its decentralization. Each consumer worries only about what goods to buy and what they cost, not how to produce them. Each supplier of a good worries only about how to produce it and what it sells for. Economists can show that under certain idealized assumptions, a market system yields highly efficient composition and distribution of output—and all without heavy-handed central planning or control. In other words, the pursuit of individual self-interest, guided only by the "invisible hand" of competition (to use Adam Smith's term), also serves the common good.

But what about fairness? Will the resulting distribution get goods to the "right" people, giving them a "fair" reward for their contribution to society? The answer depends on one's definition of fairness.

A case that the market outcome is fair can be made. When price rises to eliminate excess demand for a good, those who value the good most get it. When markets set the incomes for labor and other productive resources, those who contribute valued resources to society reap the rewards.

Of course, in a system based on fair market exchange, those who have nothing to put in get nothing out. Moreover, the initial distribution of productive resources—personal characteristics such as intelligence, beauty, and physical strength as well as ownership of land and natural resources—is heavily influenced by chance and past history. Even in a perfectly functioning market system, most people would support, on fairness grounds, some intervention to ensure that those with limited initial resources have enough purchasing power to live a decent life.

In addition, the assumptions *are* idealized, and real markets never work as well as the ideal. Nevertheless, for many economists, the virtues of the ideal, and the perception that real markets usually do perform the task of resource allocation reasonably well, set up a preference for markets. When a market does not produce the desired results, economists are inclined to look for a way to fix the market, rather than to abandon it altogether. For example, if some people lack basic necessities, their preferred solution is to redistribute income, rather than to control the prices of the needed goods or give them as handouts.

So why not let a market allocate physician services and, in the process, determine what physicians earn? Why not, indeed? Historically, this is exactly what happened. Physicians marketed their services to consumers, and each service had its price—the fee-for-service system. However, in the opinion of many observers, the market approach does not produce satisfactory results for health care.

PROBLEMS WITH THE MARKET OUTCOME

Expenditures for medical care have been rising rapidly, both in absolute amounts and as a percentage of gross national product.[1] The United States has a higher per capita GNP and spends a greater percentage of it on medical care than any other industrialized nation. Yet many Americans are concerned about whether we are getting good value for our money.

Large groups of Americans have serious difficulty obtaining and affording even routine health care. Key health statistics such as infant mortality rates are surprisingly high for an affluent, industrialized country, especially for the groups known to have poor access to care.

Even for well-insured middle-class patients, patterns of care often seem inappropriate. For example, the system seems biased toward excessive use of technology-based procedures and diagnostic tests and against cognitively based physician services, toward hospital care and away from home- and community-based care, toward care for acute illness and away from rehabilitative care, and so on.

Physician services are *not* the major component in total expenditures. Nevertheless, physicians are extremely well paid in comparison with the average person in need of medical care, or even in comparison with members of other professions requiring comparable levels of skill and specialized training. Moreover, physicians play a key role in the delivery of other health care goods and services. Thus, public attention is inevitably focused on the market for their services.

There is increasing debate about what to do. Clearly, one problem may be the failure of the physician services market to meet the assumptions of the idealized model. Note that the issue is not whether the physician services market is imperfect. All markets are a little bit imperfect. The issue is whether the market is so imperfect, or whether this good is so different from other goods, that it should be distributed by some completely different process.

There are a variety of imperfections in the physician services market one can point to, some being the consequence of deliberate government policy (for example, the restrictions on entry embodied in the licensure system). Two sources of market imperfections have been repeatedly identified as of special importance, however. These are the asymmetry in information between patient and physician and the uneven and unpredictable distribution of health needs.

IMPERFECT INFORMATION

The standard market model assumes that buyers have perfect information about the product they are buying and the utility it will yield. This is a simplification, but not a bad one in the case of most commodities.

Physician services are an exception. To decide how much utility will result from a purchase of physician services, the buyer must typically rely on the advice of the very person who will supply them. In other words, the physician acts as an *agent*, helping the patient determine what to buy.

As a result, physicians can influence the demand for health care by the advice they give. If physicians make exactly the same decisions their patients would make if they had the same medical knowledge, the agency factor does not distinguish this market from others. But do they? In fact, should they? What *is* the agent's duty—to the patient, to the rest of society, and to himself or herself? And what happens if these duties conflict?

Many of the ethical questions currently troubling physicians are related to the question of the proper nature of agency. Ethical issues in the payment of physicians are discussed in greater depth elsewhere in this book. We must touch on them here, however, because of their importance to the economic framework.

Many physicians believe it is their ethical duty as a patient's agent to do everything medically beneficial for that patient *without regard to cost*. Of course, the patient must pay the cost. A patient who cannot afford the care a physician believes is beneficial raises a difficult dilemma. If the patient is already in the physician's care, duty requires that the care be provided anyway. Physicians with too many such patients court financial disaster for themselves and their families. They must manage their practices so that they do not take on too many patients who are likely to need charity care, taking refuge in the belief that their ethical duty extends only to those patients for whom they have accepted initial responsibility.

This view of agency differs from the economist's view. Economists (and some physicians) are more inclined to see agency as a contractual relationship in which the physician undertakes to serve the patient's interest *as the patient defines it*. After all, even if a patient can find the money, the medical benefits it buys may not compensate for the sacrifices made necessary in other areas of life. In this view, a physician *should* consider cost to the extent that it matters to the patient (of course, taking care to make sure the patient fully understands the trade-offs between medical benefits and costs).

These two positions differ in their understanding of the meaning of serving a patient's interest. They are united, however, in ignoring the interests of others. The first does so on the grounds that to do otherwise is unethical; the second, on the grounds that it is unnecessary. In an idealized market system, efficiency is served by decentralization, and equity is promoted, if necessary, through policies implemented at other levels of the system—for example, through taxes and transfers of purchasing power.

UNEVEN AND UNPREDICTABLE DISTRIBUTION OF NEEDS

Neither position adequately accounts for the complications raised by the variability in health care needs. One's demands for health care depends on one's health, which in turn depends on chance. Few people have the resources to ensure access to all the important medical care they might want in all situations. Fortunately, there is a market response. For protection against the financial consequences of changes in health status, people can buy insurance.

Once a person is insured, however, the insurance company picks up at least some of the cost. Suddenly, price no longer plays its beneficial role as mediator between consumer preferences and resource costs to society. Consumers don't weigh the marginal utility of health care against the price because they do not pay the price. Of course, they pay indirectly because premiums must cover the expenditures on behalf of all those insured, but there is no incentive to consider this since any one person's consumption is just a small part of the whole.

A system of extensive health insurance in which physicians are paid on a fee-for-service basis greatly eases ethical conflicts. The more physicians do for patients, the more they are paid; yet the insurance coverage shields patients from the full financial consequences. Health insurance began with coverage of hospital care and the physician fees associated with it, the care most likely to create ethical dilemmas. This care is expensive, not within the doctor's direct financial control, and usually less discretionary than other care. Routine physician services are less well covered, but also more affordable.

In this system, the difference between the two concepts of agency blurs. Physicians are protected from worry about the adverse financial effects of clinical decisions on themselves or the rest of society as long as they minimize involvement with the uninsured and those on public programs that pay below-market fees.

EFFICIENCY IMPLICATIONS

The problem is that this world is one in which neither patient nor doctor cares about the relationship between benefits and costs. When the doctor is paid on a fee-for-service basis and the patient is well insured, both are happy to use medical care to the point where further care would yield no benefits at all, rather than stopping at a point where benefits are commensurate with costs. Thus, many people are getting care that is not worth what it costs.

Under these conditions, there is also little pressure on suppliers to produce efficiently. In a competitive market the pressure of competition *makes* producers stay efficient. If they do not, they are put out of business by the competition. Physicians can make more money if they use inputs (including their own time) as efficiently as possible, but they do not have to, to stay in business. This is one reason why so little is known about the trade-offs between costs and health benefits.

Recent work by William Hsiao and his colleagues[2] underscores the extent to which the price system is not playing its normal role in the physician services market. These researchers show that the relative prices of individual services do not reflect relative resource inputs. Similarly, the returns to different medical specialties do not correspond appropriately to either the investment in specialized training or the difficulty of the work. Their work also suggests (more indirectly) that prices also do not reflect the relative values that consumers place on the services.

Market organization without a price system or some functional substitute for it leads to a situation of rising costs and insurance premiums, even as the well insured receive a pattern of care that fails to match benefits with costs. Millions of people cannot afford private insurance, but are not eligible for public insurance; yet a major obstacle to expanded public coverage is the public sense that such an expansion would be extremely expensive for the benefits secured.

What to do? First, it is important to reach a new consensus on the role of the physician. In a world of third-party payment, an economist would argue that the concept of agency must be understood in a broader sense. A narrow definition of self-interest seems to lead a patient to prefer a doctor whose clinical decisions ignore all costs that do not fall directly on the patient. Yet the patient is part of a risk pool that in the aggregate bears the costs of all care received by the members. It is in the patient's long-term interest to agree to limits on utilization that reflect an evaluation of the relative benefits and costs of treatments. This holds down the cost of membership in the risk pool and ensures that the common resources are not squandered on low- or zero-benefit care. Similarly, the definition of the physician's ethical duty as one of pure patient advocacy without regard to consequences for others seems too narrow, given the interconnected dependence we have on one another for health care resources.

These are arguments based on efficiency considerations. The point is that unless this interconnectedness is taken into account by physicians, we will spend too much for the advantages of risk pooling. These arguments arise even in the absence of disparities in purchasing power that make it difficult for people to afford insurance or disparities in initial health status that make insurers reluctant to offer insurance to poor risks at reasonable prices.

EQUITY IMPLICATIONS

When fairness considerations are added as well, the arguments become stronger. Economists begin with a preference for handling equity with transfers of purchasing power. A more rational and generous income redistribution policy would certainly be a useful step toward improving access to health care for those who now lack it. Nevertheless, it would be unlikely to solve the problem entirely, given the limits of private insurance markets in pooling the risks resulting from genetic health endowments and chronic illness. Moreover, society seems to prefer a more direct approach to redistribution of health care. Given this, a system that gets benefits in line with costs will also make tax dollars go farther in the purchase of health benefits for the disadvantaged.

REMEDIES

One approach often advocated by economists is to bring financial incentives back into the patient's decisions to use care, by moving away from first dollar coverage and introducing more cost sharing at the point of use. This approach is helpful, but inherently limited. Cost sharing cannot go very far without losing the very thing people seek in pooling their risk— freedom from the worry of unexpected large medical bills. Moreover, patients still need to rely on their physicians for advice about the benefits of care.

Information asymmetries, the need for risk pooling, and the special redistributive importance of medical care mean that we cannot rely on a decentralized market process to produce an efficient and equitable allocation of health care at the individual patient level. Mechanisms must be found to do what prices do in simpler markets.

Inevitably, physicians must play a central role. The system must somehow guide doctors to practice cost-conscious medicine—cost conscious in the sense that patients get neither too much *nor* too little in terms of either quantity or quality of care.

The task is enormously difficult. Not only is medical care complex, but also individual preferences differ. Care that some patients consider highly beneficial and want desperately is care that others do not want and consider harmful. An acceptable system must take account of the complexity of medical technology and the complexity of individual values.

It is probably impossible to do what needs to be done purely through financial incentives to physicians. A successful approach will require a combination of financial incentives, ethical principles, and explicit guidance (e.g., through standards of practice set by the profession and the public and private third-party payers working together in the public interest, quality assurance activities, and so on). A balance will have to be sought between two unpleasant extremes, sometimes pejoratively described as individual physicians "practicing cost-benefit analysis at the bedside" or, alternatively, "practicing cookbook medicine out of government cookbooks."

It is essential, however, that the overall thrust of the system of financial rewards to physicians be in harmony with society's concept of their role in the allocation of resources. This chapter has described the underlying goals of a physician payment system and explained why the usual methods do not produce satisfactory results. The chapters that follow discuss specific methods of physician payment currently in place or under consideration.

NOTES

1. These issues are discussed in many articles and books. The seminal article in health economics is K. J. Arrow, "Uncertainty and the Welfare Economics of Medical Care," *American Economic Review* 53 (1963): 941–69. One comprehensive overview of current issues in health economics is P. Feldstein, *Health Care Economics*, 3d ed. (New York: Wiley, 1988). See also M. A. Baily, "The Word 'Rationing' and American Health Policy," *Journal of Health Politics and Law* 9 (1984): 489–501; and M. A. Baily, "Rationing Medical Care: Processes for Defining Adequacy," in G. J. Agich and C. E. Begley, eds., *The Price of Health* (Dordrecht, Holland: Reidel, 1986).

2. W. C. Hsiao et al., "Estimating Physicians' Work for a Resource-Based Relative-Value Scale," *New England Journal of Medicine* 319 (1988): 835–41. W. C. Hsiao et al., "Results and Policy Implications of the Resource-Based Relative-Value Study," *New England Journal of Medicine* 319 (1988): 881–88.

Part II

Assessing Payment Mechanisms

In this section we will make the transition from analytic frameworks to descriptions and critical assessments of physician payment mechanisms. Robert A. Berenson reviews specific payment methods (fee-for-service, prospective payment, and capitation) and their implications for cost containment. Steven R. Eastaugh places these methods in the context of related issues such as physician supply, appropriate practice guidelines, physician service volume, and workload scales before turning to four reform ideas. These commentaries make clear the current preference for some capitated means of reform.

In a lively discussion of the role of high-technology medicine in physician reimbursement issues, Richard K. Riegelman adds uncertainty, income concerns, and liability to a potent formula that drives up the costs of care and resists efforts to control it. He argues that reformed professional standards rather than structural techniques such as capitation will ultimately be applied to control costs in an era when both patients and providers are fascinated by technology. Finally, John E. Ott projects a new form of organization for health care delivery, one he calls competitive medical organizations (CMOs). An alternative to some form of national health insurance, the CMO would be cost effective, Ott argues, because it will be based on profits that will be distributed based on efficient and effective care rather than by cost shifting.

Of course, reform of the way doctors are paid relates to the way the medical system works or fails to work. As one reads the chapters in this part, it is worth keeping in mind that there are three general reform strategies: rationing, removing, and redesigning.

When a commodity is limited, we find ways to ration it, which is really a form of allocation. Pricing is a type of rationing that relates to at least some medical care, such as cosmetic surgery. Another method of rationing health care resources is the line, the "queue," which has especially been used in Great Britain. A particularly American way to ration, one that might be called rationing by fine print, relies on the difference between the consumer's expectation and the system's reality. For example, when it is said that all "indicated" or "necessary" care will be offered, these terms might conceal a difference between what might be offered and what is in fact available.

Another method for dealing with cost is removing the problem, thus effectively shifting it to someone else. This occurred in the past when some emergency rooms reallocated the uninsured patient load by sending them to county hospitals. In recent years Medicare rules have emphasized shifting the costs of medical care to the patient and to other insurance plans. Insurance plans not only may shift costs by transferring financial burdens to others, but also may "skim" by enrolling the healthiest patients in order to minimize the costs of getting reimbursed for their medical care.

A third reform option is to redesign the system by considering who, when, where, and how services are offered. The expanded use of allied health professionals, clinics in nontraditional sites like the work place and shopping centers, prevention rather than acute intervention, and how technology is used are all subjects that have to do with redesign. As the next few chapters will make clear, our health care system is ripe for creative approaches to reform.

5

Financial Methods for Paying the Doctor: Issues and Options

Steven R. Eastaugh

Concerning the coming surplus of 60,000 physicians, I use "surplus" with caution because I do not believe the United States will ever see a surplus such as exists in some Western European countries, where trained physicians have taken jobs as taxicab drivers and have applied for welfare.
>   —Alvin Tarlov, M.D., Chairman of the 1981 Graduate Medical
>   Education National Advisory Committee[1]

Our current problems are also our past solutions.
>   —John D. Thompson

Since the publication of the Tarlov GMENAC study in 1981 the concept of a doctor glut (oversupply) has become part of the conventional wisdom. In the context of the 1990s the term *glut* might be a misnomer, like the term *doctor shortage* in the 1960s. In his classic book *The Doctor Shortage*, Rashi Fein points to the two real problems: maldistribution of physician supply by geographic location and by specialty choice (i.e., too many specialists).[2] As a number of economists from the Rand Corporation have most recently pointed out, this maldistribution problem has been diminished as the supply of physicians per capita has increased. However, perception of a glut of doctors is still the conventional wisdom among policymakers, regardless of the data.

A number of so-called procompetition measures were initiated in the 1980s to stimulate cost-decreasing behavior. In reaction to regulations and payer-driven fee negotiations, the physician community has been more willing to accept utilization review programs and discount pricing because of the so-called "doctor glut."[3] Consequently, the perceived doctor glut has served as a primary catalyst for change in payment policies even if the projected oversupply of 60,000 physicians in ten to twenty years never becomes a reality. The GMENAC study overestimated supply, as fewer doctors are being trained and clinicians are spending fewer hours each month on patient care.[4] A recent study by Schwartz, Sloan, and Mendelson[5] suggests that a slight shortage of physicians might exist by the year 2000 if the capitated health plans (health maintenance organizations, preferred provider organizations, and other managed care plans[6]) do not achieve a 28 percent market share of the American population. Such predictions of a 30,000-physician shortage due to AIDS and inefficient fee-for-service medical staffing ratios are highly suspect, as the Schwartz study concedes. Demand-expanding and demand-constraining forces flow like a tide over a medical community hardly conscious of economic forces. Technological change could increase patient demand beyond all projections, whereas corporate and federal attempts to ration services could decrease the demand for physician services. Whether society has an under- or oversupply of doctors depends on two factors: demand (highly unpredictable) and supply (stable in the 1990s compared to the rapid growth era in the period 1965–1982).

RECENT TRENDS IN PHYSICIAN SUPPLY

In 1978 medical schools received over 45,000 applications. By 1988 the number of applications for 16,400 medical school slots had declined to under 24,000, and many of the applicants were multiple reapplicants. The demand for medical education had declined by 50 percent in one decade. The reasons that fewer students are applying to medical school are complex. While physicians are fighting to maintain their authority and their income, third-party payers are attempting to constrain prices and volume levels. These payers are implementing peer review programs to affect the style of medical care and are having some sentinel effect in determining unnecessary or inappropriate medical care.[7] It is ironic that in countries where doctors have economic freedom (e.g., where they are not salaried employees of a public system) they practice medicine with less clinical freedom.[8] Cost containment has replaced the cost-is-no-concern view of medical practice in America.

The data in Table 5.1 from the American Medical Association survey for *Physician Characteristics and Distribution* (hereafter referred to as AMA survey) indicate recent trends in physician supply. One can observe in the second line the steady climb in the supply of physicians per capita. A geographic maldistribution of physicians still exists beyond what can be expected from trends in urban group practice and from the perceived need to create citadels for medical education in urban centers. New York State is still 44 percent above the national average of physicians per capita, and

Table 5.1
Supply of Allopathic M.D.s and M.D. Characteristics, 1963–2000[a]

	1963	1970	1980	1985	1990[b]	2000[b]
Number of active M.D.s	258,958	314,217	440,357	512,849	568,000	664,000
M.D.s per 100,000 population[c]	135	151	189	211	227	248
M.D.s per 100,000 population:						
General & family practice		27.8	26.0	27.6	28.7	26
Internal medicine		20.1	30.9	37.2	42.4	49
Other medical specialty		17.0	23.5	28.5	34.3	38
Surgical specialties		41.3	47.9	52.8	58.6	69
Anesthesiology		5.2	6.9	9.1	11.0	13
Psychiatry[d]		11.2	13.4	14.9	16.0	19
Radiology		6.4	8.8	10.4	10.2	10
Other specialties		21.6	31.1	30.1	26.2	24
Major locus of activity as a percentage of active M.D.s:						
Office-based		57.6%	58.2%	59.7%	58.9%	57%
Hospital-based		25.8	22.3	21.5	20.2	19
Teaching/research/admin.		9.7	8.2	8.7	9.3	12
Other activities		6.8	11.2	10.1	11.5	12
Percentage of foreign medical graduates (FMGs)	13%	20%	23%	22%	21%	18%
FMGs as a percentage of residents	28%	33%	25%	16%	13%	11%

[a]These figures do not include osteopathic doctors (D.O.s): 12,000 in 1970; 17,100 in 1980; 22,000 in 1985; 28,000 in 1990; 40,000 in 2000.

[b]1990 and 2000 estimates by the author.

[c]Inactive M.D.s vary from 19,000 to 39,000 depending on the AMA survey year for *Physician Characteristics and Distribution.*

[d]Psychiatry includes child psychiatry.

Mississippi is 37 percent below average physician supply. Some of the growth in physician supply ratio is necessary due to the aging of the population, but some of the additional physicians specialize in quality-of-life subspecialty care (e.g., plastic surgery).[9, 10] A very slight tendency toward more primary care physicians has been observed. In the 1980s the supply of primary care physicians grew faster than that of all nonprimary care physicians (30 percent compared to 23 percent) (AMA survey). The primary locus for physician activity seems to change at a glacial pace toward more administration and research activity and less office-based, fee-for-service self-employment. Those who think that office-based practitioners will in the future decline at a faster pace should reflect on the 1910 Flexner Report. Those who predicted the demise of the private practitioner following publication of the 1910 report were grossly inaccurate.[11]

One last trend apparent in Table 5.1 is the decline in foreign medical graduates (FMGs) since the mid-1980s after Congress took action to restrict the flow of immigrant physicians. Public hospitals and small marginal teaching hospitals are still highly dependent on an FMG work force to deliver patient care.[10]

One educational response to the perceived doctor glut in the 1980s has been to lengthen the period of graduate medical education. For example, plastic surgery residents spent 50 percent more time in graduate training in 1989 than they did in 1981. Their elder senior medical staff may lengthen the apprenticeship to enhance the quality of care and also possibly to keep their competition in the educational pipeline for as long as possible. On a national average, 38 percent of the physicians who will be in practice in 1999 are in training in 1990 (AMA survey). Some of the younger doctors in training wish their elders would listen to Hippocrates and reflect that "the life is so short and the craft so long to learn." Lucky Hippocrates never faced a $50,000 debt service from his medical education.

A career in medicine is being viewed as increasingly regulated and less profitable, compared to prior decades. According to the AMA survey of socioeconomic characteristics of medical practice, physician incomes after inflation increased only a total of 5.4 percent from 1979 to 1988. However, the average medical school tuition outpaced inflation by 194 percent over the decade. Those without substantial wealth have to incur a sizable debt before graduation day. Nearly one in every four graduates was more than $50,000 in debt by graduation. Because of the proliferation of bureaucratic paperwork and the increasing competition within the profession, some doctors are steering young people away from a career in medicine.

Clearly nonfinancial factors such as loss of autonomy and prestige contribute to the downward trend in applications to medical school. Medicine is not a poverty profession. As an index of physicians' economic status within a society one can consider the ratio of physicians' net income to gross domestic product per capita within a nation. In 1988 by that yardstick the West German physician outpaced the general public in his or her country by a ratio of 7.2:1, closely followed by American and Japanese physicians (6.6:1).[12] However, these pretax medical practice figures understate the economic advantage among Japanese physicians, who have such high status that by law they pay no income taxes. In contrast, the physicians in most of Western Europe outpace the general public by 3.9 to 4.2. Because of the high tax rates in those countries with national health insurance, it is futile to negotiate higher salaries, so the clinicians negotiate about working hours and working conditions.[13]

While American physicians fear the idea of government-negotiated salaries, the cost escalation problem is driving Congress to consider broad systemic reforms in the payment of physicians. In 1989 physicians' income represented 23 percent of personal health expenditures and 2.24 percent of the gross national product. If unconstrained, physician expenses will rise to $1,400 per capita by the year 2000. This brief chapter cannot survey all physician manpower issues, but many analysts believe there is a maldistribution of types of physician (too many surgeons and subspecialists, not enough primary care or internal medicine specialists). However, some economic analysis suggests that even in the year 2000 some large cities will have a deficit of most types of subspecialists.[14] Before surveying the payment options, one should survey the incentives implicit in the three basic methods of paying the doctor.

PRINCIPLE METHODS FOR PAYING THE DOCTOR

The three basic methods for compensating clinicians are salary, capitation, and fee-for-service. Each method has relative strengths and weaknesses. (For a more extended discussion of these methods see Chapter 6.)

The primary advantages of a salaried system are cost control and a controlled workweek (many young doctors like the life-style advantage of working a salaried shift and going home). If a doctor is salaried, paid per unit of time, the organizational risk involves poor productivity and potential underprovision of care. The salaried individual can try to come late and leave early and try to do a minimum amount of work per hour. Because of this obvious moral hazard to underprovide service, salaried physician contracts increasingly include an incentive compensation provision to pay more for enhanced productivity. Clever salaried physician contracts try to promote the carrot (additional pay for additional work above the average), rather than emphasizing the stick (sanctions if one fails to meet a workload quota).

The second method for paying physicians involves capitation. Pure capitation pays the doctor a fixed payment per person joining his or her panel of potential patients. The incentives are to keep the patient happy and healthy (happy so they do not disenroll and healthy so they do not overutilize expensive health care resources). Capitation offers no incentive to over-provide expensive care, and it offers the long-term incentive to provide preventive care (thus saving money in future years). In our mobile American society, this last incentive is probably overstated because subscribers change jobs and health plans often; thus, the capitated system providing the preventive care accrues a small fraction of the financial benefits. Capitated, managed care systems make the doctor a gatekeeper, with the dual responsibilities to do no harm to the patient while acting as an explicit guardian of the health plan's financial welfare. Capitated systems run the risk of undercare, so quality must be closely monitored. Capitated systems also run the risk of overreferral, in that gatekeepers may minimize their workload by shunting too many patients to specialists elsewhere in the health plan (this can be controlled through the process of utilization review and reinforced through financial incentives by providing less holdout pay at year's end). A number of managed care systems have demonstrated that physicians can practice excellent and cost-effective medicine under a capitated contract. Unnecessary admissions and routine tests (e.g., chest roentgenograms) can be reduced without detriment to the patient. Consequently, capitated payment is the most rapidly growing method of paying physicians in the 1980s.

The predominant, but declining, method for paying the doctor is fee-for-service.[15] Under fee-for-service payment per unit of work, the clinician's income is directly related to work ethic and business acumen. However, just as capitation runs the potential risk of conflict of interest for financial reasons, fee-for-service offers the conflict of interest to steer patients to tests or facilities in which the doctor reaps financial returns (e.g., because he or she owns the equipment that does the test or receives kickback incentive pay for referrals). It looks greedy to the public if the clinician is a business partner with the laboratory and the radiology imaging center. In fact, Congress is increasingly wary of the argument that the physician is unconcerned with cash flow and owns such facilities only to ensure the quality of patient care. Fee-for-service doctors get paid more if they provide more services, but they also get paid more (1) if they are paid as the owners of the equipment that does the test or procedure and then paid again to interpret the results, and (2) if they are paid for upcoding (upgrading) the coded work done to receive higher payment rates. The fee-for-service system has been very inflationary because all the incentives stimulate overprovision of inappropriate or unnecessary care. In contrast, salaried or capitated physicians have no incentive to own health care facilities or to upcode the patient record.[10]

WANTED: SOME EFFECTIVE CONTROLS ON QUANTITY AND QUALITY

Capitation systems are growing in popularity because governments and insurance companies want to negotiate with bundles of services, fewer sellers, and risk-contracting care organizations (i.e., a few hundred plans willing to take an annual per-person check as payment in full). In terms of both cost control and administrative simplicity, capitated plans are superior to dealing separately with 500,000 physicians and each and every ancillary service provider and their unbundled pile of bills. However, organized medicine fears declining professional autonomy and the prerogative to exceed the employer's norms for standard care if clinicians are only salaried or capitated employees of some faceless corporation. A change in physician attitudes may emerge over the 1990s as guidelines and models are developed for plans that have excellent quality as well as excellent cost-efficiency. Billions of dollars could be saved each year if physicians practiced in the style of those at Stanford, or the Mayo Clinic, or Case Western Reserve. [7, 9, 16, 17] Such facilities are what John E. Ott (see Chapter 8) refers to as competitive medical organizations (CMOs), which act as islands for the 5 to 20 percent of the physicians in an area who enhance quality, take responsibility for patient needs, and make prudent decisions concerning discretionary care.

Naive policymakers question the concept of discretionary care, saying that the world is black or white and care is either unnecessary or necessary, and that there is no middle category. One could expand Ott's concept of the CMO one step further and suggest that such organizations represent pathway guidelines for better medical practice at a reasonable cost in the community. Pathway guidelines serve as yardsticks for cost-effective clinical decision making[18] and as standards to demonstrate that good medicine and good economics can coexist.[19] Too much attention has been focused on a second type of guideline: boundary guidelines used by payers to define the range of medical practice and beyond which a clinician incurs the wrath of the payers. If the practitioner exceeds the boundary, the computer suggests an administrative sanction, and after a number of due process hearings, a monetary penalty may result. This second type of guideline gives the topic a bad reputation and has lead to the phrase "cookbook medicine." Physicians are not ignorant or venal, but many clinicians need help with the positive, proactive type of pathway guideline. If physicians wish to preserve their autonomy, they should actively participate in the development of pathway guidelines. Case management can remain a caring art, and not a cold cookbook formula, if beacons are developed to assist experienced practitioners in developing pathway guidelines. The guidelines are suggestions, and the microcomputer is more of an educational tool than an enemy to be consorted with as a part of standard federal operating procedure.[20] In summary, boundary guidelines clamp down on "bad" physicians, whereas pathway guidelines assist the profession.

What constitutes appropriate care and an optimal pathway can be established in three basic ways: the implicit ad hoc method, the risk-benefit method, and the cost-benefit method. Decision trees in academic settings focus on the cost-benefit method (an action is appropriate if the marginal benefit exceeds the marginal cost, with the intangible benefits shadow priced). The risk-benefit approach suffers because this method includes only traditional medical risks and excludes monetary costs. The implicit approach used in hospital utilization review is hard to export to other settings and has questionable validity, given that we know little of what the reviewer had in mind during the ad hoc process of making judgments.[7, 9, 21, 22, 23]

CONTROLLING THE VOLUME OF SERVICES

The great equation in medical economics involves the control of expenditures (E) which equal price (P) times quantity (Q). All payers desire to control E by trimming P and constraining Q. The health care system is a very adaptable balloon: Squeezing down on only one factor (e.g., P) can come out in another area (e.g., increased Q). Medicare Part B services, which pay for physician services, averaged an 18.7 percent annual increase from 1975 to 1984 until Congress imposed a price freeze in 1984. During the first year of the freeze the growth rate declined to 8.3 percent per year, but rebounded to 16.2 percent in 1985 and 14.3 percent in 1986. The price freeze was coopted by an obvious expansion in volume. Congress lifted the freeze as part of the October 1986 Omnibus Reconciliation Act.[10] However, in the thirty months following the lifting of the fee freeze the Part B expenditures per capita increased 17 percent per annum, while prices rose only an average of 2.4 percent.[15] Price controls without volume controls yield little in the way of cost control, and service volume per capita is clearly out of control. Physicians can expand volume by a stepped-up quantity of procedures, operations, and provider-initiated follow-up visits. Moreover, with 7,200 codes available to label physician services, including six subjective codes for the basic office visit, code creep (upcoding) becomes prevalent. The fine detail of the codes allows the smart physician to unbundle the patient experience or upcode individual items (e.g., the minimal visit is upcoded as brief, and the extended visit is upcoded as a comprehensive office visit). Hospitals have played the same game in the 1980s with diagnosis-related groups (DRGs) as patient classifications creep to the better-paying, higher-code groups.

Some of the added volume and intensity might represent real health benefits to patients, but some of the increase has been clearly labeled unnecessary and inappropriate by the federal Health Care Financing Administration (HCFA).[24] The number one physician reimbursement issue seems to involve controlling the growth in per capita service volume. The most effective single solution is capitation. Capitation decentralizes decisions about which patient receives what and how much, while heightening the need for quality assurance and minimizing the chance of underprovision of care. Capitation will not be the voluntary choice of all Americans, as evidenced by the fact that capitated Medicare covers only 1.4 million Americans. Since 1988

HCFA has pilot-tested an improved average adjusted per capita cost (AAPCC) formula in six health maintenance organizations (HMOs), using a health status adjustment factor based on demographic data to place individuals in diagnostic cost groups (DCGs).[25] A ratebook has been established by which enrollees will be classified in a particular cost weight category based on age, sex, welfare status, and the highest number of eight possible DCGs associated with a hospitalization in the previous fifteen months (DCG 0 = no hospitalization or a discretionary 1- or 2-day hospitalization). Ash and Ellis[24] argue that DCGs may eliminate any incentive that exists for discouraging sick enrollees from joining a capitated plan. Capitation cures the incentive to game the payment system through an increased volume of unneccessary services and will leave the plan with the discretion for dividing the annual payments among the various physicians and facilities.

The number two physician reimbursement issue involves selecting a fair workload scale for equitable payment among physician specialties. William Hsiao and his colleagues[26, 27] worked for five years to develop a resource-based relative-value scale (RBRVS) as an alternative to the current charge-based system. Resource inputs by physicians include (1) total work input performed by the physician for each service, (2) practice costs (including office overhead and malpractice premiums), and (3) specialty training costs (e.g., the opportunity costs associated with spending thirteen years going to medical school and training to become a cardiac surgeon). The Hsiao study, with the help of the AMA and a number of specialty societies, presents fairly valid and reliable estimates of physicians' work according to four dimensions: time, psychological stress, mental effort and judgment, and technical skill plus physical effort.

The Hsiao study has been subject to one minor and one major criticism. The minor point revolves around the heavy emphasis on time measurement. Other professionals (e.g., lawyers) do not have their charges related so fully to their work time expended. This minor point is easily dismissed: (1) In the name of scientific accuracy the RBRVS is better than perpetuating tradition, (2) time orientation may stimulate physicians to enhance productivity, and (3) other professions make less use of government funds and insurance dollars (e.g., if we had government paying half the legal fees, then an RBRVS would be necessary for that profession). On a more important point, the RBRVS study methodology could be improved if a refined estimate for health status improvement to the patient could become a major measure of workload. Hsiao could only equate physician activity with workload. If activity were replaced by health status improvement as the purists' measure for effective workload, the providers who offer better care could be paid better. In the business world this mechanism would be labeled pay-for-performance.[28] Obviously, not all activity proves to be beneficial, given that the real output in an ideal study would be health status improvement. If

Table 5.2
Physicians' Charges and Workload Under a Resource-Based Relative-Value Scale
(RBRVS)

Service Workload	Charge (1987)	Work Units	Charge per Work Unit
Follow-up visit of family physician to nursing home patient, with extended service	$ 37	159	$0.23
Diagnostic proctosigmoidoscopy examination of colon	53	118	0.45
Simple repair of superficial wound, 2.5 to 7.5 cm	66	75	0.88
Delivery of child (vaginal)	481	407	1.18
Repair of inguinal hernia (in the groin)	732	476	1.54
Triple coronary artery bypass	4,663	2,871	1.62
Insertion of permanent pacemaker (ventricular)	1,440	620	2.32

we had a refined health status measure, the clinicians who produce higher-quality patient outcomes could get paid more for their effort and skill.[10, 19]

The basic research question the Hsiao study answers is how much to pay for cognitive services related to procedures. The present payment system is biased toward paying for procedures done to the patient, rather than for talking to or thinking about the patient. The specialist who spends fifteen minutes inserting a Swan Ganz catheter into a patient who has heart failure receives $175, but the doctor who spends forty minutes doing a history and physical on the same patient arrives at the diagnosis and is paid only $70.[29] Under the Hsiao scheme, physicians would be paid more equitably per unit of work (there would not be a tenfold variation in the last column of Table 5.2). If the gains and losses to physicians were redistributed in a zero sum fashion between the various specialties, $140,000 of income would be carved out of the average thoracic surgeon's $350,000 in 1988. Most surgeons would lose money, but urologists and otolaryngologists would lose only a fraction. Primary care fees would rise by more than 60 percent, which might (1) cause physicians to spend more time talking with their patients and (2) re-energize the declining supply of filled residency positions in internal medicine (many medical programs have gone begging for residents since 1986).

Surgeons and other specialty groups most affected by the Hsiao study suggest that redistribution of physician fees could worsen the volume of services (e.g., more discretionary operations might be performed, and not be detected by peer review or second opinion surgery programs). In a pessimistic worst case scenario the RBRVS would not stimulate many more primary care doctors to accept assignment under Medicare and the government check as payment, but a massive number of surgeons already on assignment with Medicare (because surgical fees are difficult to collect) would either drop assignment (and charge more) or drop out of the Medicare program.[15] This scare scenario seems unlikely because surgeons are in need of the cash flow. From 1979 to 1988 the number of surgeons has increased from 8,514 to over 12,000, but the average number of operations per surgeon declined 26 percent (thus proving that supply and demand are alive and well in the surgical marketplace) (AMA survey). Surgeons need Medicare business too much to drop out of the Medicare program. Moreover, HCFA never hoped that an RBRVS scheme would induce a flood of demand for primary care by the elderly, given the tight budgets.

The importance of the Hsiao study is not simply as a cost control mechanism to keep the FY 1992 Medicare budget from exceeding $124 billion. The RBRVS will give all payers a device by which to implement a type of aggressive price competition unknown to physicians. Each insurance company could go to the medical community and ask for a single number, on a sealed bid, for their minimum-contract-price relative-value multiplier. Insurance companies would then have a simple device, and one confidential number on a piece of paper, to force physicians to bid down their prices (and incomes) each year.

ALTERNATIVES TO "OVERHAUL GRADUALLY"

The phrase "overhaul gradually" is a classic oxymoron, two words that do not go together. We know we need major changes (overhaul), but the process will be gradual and multiyear. Yet we know that the physician community will resist major changes in payment policies, even as we know that the policy must be dramatic to curtail a 17 percent inflation rate in Medicare Part B expenditures.[28] A number of alternatives, not all mutually exclusive, have been suggested. One could simply reform the existing system to prevent upcoding by reducing the number of available billing codes. This idea worked in the Canadian context with Quebec physicians, but may not prove as effective with American doctors who see their incomes protected by code-creeping the seldom audited patient code conditions or procedures into better-paying classification categories.

The second reform idea, fee schedules, involves implementing the Hsiao RBRVS concept such that a uniform price list dictates the same pay rate for similar services. (This is in marked contrast to uniform customary rates that have wide variability.)

A third reform idea, payment for packages of services, sets a prospective rate that puts doctors at financial risk for the use and cost of those services.[30] For example, the DRG prices could be expanded to include physician fees (e.g., if the care is done more efficiently, the physician receives a higher residual share of the check, and the payer provides extra outlier payments for severely ill patients). Ambulatory care could be reimbursed through an analogous DRG mechanism of ambulatory visit groups (AVGs).[31] The problem with the third reform idea is that it may fall prey to the law of small numbers. Consider the use of DRGs to pay hospitals. Hospitals are partly protected from undue financial risk by the effect of large numbers, if each DRG has more than seventy-five to one hundred cases. But individual physicians may have only one to two patients in each category and experience a poverty wage if their patient mix is more severely ill relative to the average. AVG payments would unfairly redistribute payments from those clinicians with genuinely more complex and costly cases for a given AVG to their peers who have less complex cases.

Capitation, the fourth reform idea, is currently the most popular reform initiative. Whether the nation moves to capitation or tougher fee schedules, specialists left out in the cold are headed for two possible fates: serious financial trouble and/or membership in a union.[32, 33] As the payers get tougher with doctors, these doctors must respond with a countervailing force that acts as a bargaining unit.

JOIN TOGETHER OR SUFFER ALONE

As the AMA was formed to combat the cults in the nineteenth century, aggressive specialty unions may form in the future to defend their declining incomes and strike for better-quality patient care. Unionization, once a dirty word in the medical world, is spreading. The California-based Union of American Physicians and Dentists has twenty-nine state chapters. Politically conservative physicians may have to face two economic truths: (1) Unions are not always bad, and (2) clinicians in overdoctored locations can properly go broke. Going broke is a major cost-containment agenda item for those that pay for medical services.[34, 35] Payers report with joy that excess economic failure among doctors and hospitals will eject the pathology from the system and drive costs down. Physicians require better productivity and a voice to negotiate on their behalf.[10] If the profession does not act together as a group, and if its members continue to pursue only individual business interests, medicine will be no more protected, or respected, than a used car dealership. Likewise, those who disrespect business skills, productivity, marketing to the public, and patients' shifting tastes will face an early retirement.

NOTES

1. A Tarlov, "The Public Thoughts of a Private Foundation Leader," *Health Affairs* 7:4 (1988): 142–56.

2. R. Fein, *The Doctor Shortage* (Washington, D.C.: Brookings Institution, 1967).

3. E. Schloss, "Beyond GMENAC—Another Physician Shortage from 2010–2030?" *New England Journal of Medicine* 318:14 (1988): 920–22.

4. GMENAC, *Report of the Graduate Medical Education National Advisory Committee to the Secretary, DHHS*, GPO 1980–0–721–748/266 (Washington, D.C.: U.S. Government Printing Office, 1981).

5. W. Schwartz, F. Sloan, and D. Mendelson, "Why There Will Be Little or No Physician Surplus Between Now and the Year 2000," *New England Journal of Medicine* 318:14 (1988): 892–97.

6. A. Enthoven, "Managed Competition of Alternative Delivery Systems," *Journal of Health Politics, Policy and Law* 13:2 (1988): 305–21.

7. J. Eisenberg, *Doctors' Decisions and the Cost of Medical Practice Patterns and Ways to Change Them* (Ann Arbor, Mich.: Health Administration Press, 1986).

8. U. Reinhardt, "Resource Allocation in Health Care: The Allocation of Lifestyles to Providers," *Milbank Memorial Fund Quarterly* 65:2 (1987): 153–76.

9. S. Eastaugh, "Placing a Value on Life and Limb: The Role of the Informed Consumer," *Health Matrix* 1:1 (1983): 5–21.

10. S. Eastaugh, *Financing Health Care: Economic Efficiency and Equity* (Dover, Mass.: Auburn House, 1987), p. 720.

11. P. Starr, *The Social Transformation of Medicine* (New York: Basic Books, 1982).

12. BASYS: 1989, *Wirkungen von Verguetungssystemen aud die Einkommen der Aerzte, die Preise und auf die Struktur aerzlicher Leistungen im Internationalen Ergleich* (Augsburg, Bavaria, West Germany: BASYS GmbH 1989, Mimeograph).

13. S. Eastaugh, *Medical Economics and Health Finance* (Dover, Mass.: Auburn House, 1981).

14. W. Schwartz, A. Williams, J. Newhouse, and C. Witsberger, "Are We Training Too Many Medical Subspecialists?" *Journal of the American Medical Association* 259:2 (1988): 233–39.

15. J. Iglehart, "Payment of Physicians Under Medicare," *New England Journal of Medicine* 318:13 (1988): 863–68.

16. P. Caper, "Solving the Medical Care Dilemma," *New England Journal of Medicine* 318:23 (1988): 1535–36.

17. D. Neuhauser, "The Quality of Medical Care and the 14 Points of Edward Deming," *Health Matrix* 6:2 (1988): 7–10.

18. S. Eastaugh, "Teaching the Principles of Cost-Effective Clinical Decision-Making to Medical Students," *Inquiry* 18:1 (1981): 28–36.

19. S. Eastaugh and J. Eastaugh, "Prospective Payment System: Further Steps to

Enhance Quality, Efficiency and Regionalization," *Health Care Management Review* 11:4 (1986): 37–52.

20. R. Derzon, "The Odd Couple in Distress: Hospitals and Physicians Face the 1990s," *Frontiers of Health Services Management* 4:3 (1988): 4–18.

21. M. Chassin, J. Kosecoff, R. Park, and R. Brook, "Does Inappropriate Use Explain Geographic Variations in the Use of Health Care Services? A Study of Three Procedures," *Journal of the American Medical Association* 258:26 (1987): 2533–37.

22. J. Wennberg, "Improving the Medical Decision-Making Process," *Health Affairs* 7:2 (1988): 99–106.

23. J. Nyman, R. Feldman, J. Shapiro, C. Grogan, and D. Link, "Changing Physician Behavior: Does Medical Review of Part B Medicare Claims Make a Difference?" *Inquiry* 27:2 (Summer 1990): 127–37.

24. A. Ash and R. Ellis, "The Diagnostic Cost Group (DCG) Methodology," (Speech presented at the 116th annual meeting of the American Public Health Association, Boston, November 15, 1988).

25. W. Hsiao et al., "Estimating Physicians' Work for a Resource-Based Relative-Value Scale," *New England Journal of Medicine* 319:13 (1988): 835–41.

26. S. Eastaugh, "Improving Productivity Under PPS: Managing Cost Reductions Without Harming Service Quality or Access," *Hospital and Health Services Administration* 30:4 (1985): 97–111.

27. E. Belker, D. Dunn, P. Braun, and W. Hsiao, "Refinement and Expansion of the Harvard Resource-Based Relative Value Scale: The Second Phase," *American Journal of Public Health* 80:7 (July 1990): 799–803.

28. Prospective Payment Assessment Commission, *Impact of the Prospective Payment System on the American Healthcare System*, ProPAC Report to Congress (Washington, D.C.: U.S. Government Printing Office, 1989).

29. J. Mitchell, "Physician DRGs," *New England Journal of Medicine* 313:11 (1985): 670–75.

30. W. Hsiao, P. Braun, D. Dunn, and E. Becker, "Resource-based Relative Value Scale," *Journal of the American Medical Association* 260:16 (October 28, 1988): 2347–2438.

31. J. Lion, M. Henderson, A. Malbon, M. Wiley, and J. Noble, "Ambulatory Visit Groups (AVGs): A Prospective Payment System for Outpatient Care," in N. Goldfield and S. Goldsmith, eds., *Financial Management of Ambulatory Care* (Rockville, Md.: Aspen, 1985), pp. 3–18.

32. S. Eastaugh, "Financing the Correct Rate of Growth of Medical Technology," *Quarterly Review of Economics and Business* 30:4 (1990): 111–23.

33. W. Glaser, "Designing Fee Schedules by Formula, Politics, and Negotiations," *American Journal of Public Health* 80:7 (July 1990): 804–9.

34. S. Eastaugh, "Universal Health Insurance: Equivocation Throughout the Nation," *New England Journal of Medicine* 322:17 (April 26, 1990): 1240.

35. G. Pope, "Physician Inputs, Outputs, and Productivity," *Inquiry* 27:2 (Summer 1990): 151–60.

6

Payment Approaches and the Cost of Care

Robert A. Berenson

Physicians in the United States receive compensation for their services in various ways: traditional fee-for-service where physicians set their charges; fee-for-service based on a uniform schedule of allowances; prepayment, including capitation; and salary. The particular payment method used has traditionally been dependent on the organizational setting in which the physician works. For example, the physician who practices individually or in a small group has been a fee-for-service provider. Large, prepaid group practices have hired physicians to work full time in their clinics.

In recent years, with increasing competition in the health care sector and the development of managed care concepts, there as been some blurring in the association between organizational setting and payment method. Group practices may give salaried M.D.s bonuses for achieving certain efficiency objectives. Open-panel health maintenance organizations (HMOs) may choose to pay either fee-for-service or capitation to contracting physicians. Whether fee-for-service or capitation, the HMO payment method may include financial risk provisions such that physicians do better or worse based on individual or group performance.

Across the board, payers and insurers in both the public and the private sectors are applying new compensation approaches that attempt to give physicians incentives to reduce marginal services and improve efficiency. Even in Great Britain, the Thatcher government has proposed modifying traditional capitation payments to general practitioners to foster competition incentives.[1] The pressure for changing the methods of compensating physicians derives mostly from unprecedented increases in spending for physician services. In 1987 payments for physician services in the United States totaled $102.7 billion, over 2 percent of the gross national product and just over 20 percent of total health spending in the country.[2] Of concern is the fact that expenditures for physician services are increasing faster than those for other health services are. For example, while expenditures for hospital care increased at an annual rate of 7.6 percent from 1982 to 1987, expenditures for physician services increased by 10.7 percent.[2] Using diagnosis-related groups (DRGs) and utilization management techniques such as prehospital authorization, third-party payers have some ability to control hospital spending. Payers are still groping for comparable techniques to moderate the rates of increase in outpatient spending, mostly for physician services.

This chapter will consider the various physician compensation models to assess how they support the goal of cost restraint, while speculating on the possible impact of these methods on the quality of care provided and on patient satisfaction. Emphasis will be given to how the impact of a particular physician payment method depends on the organizational setting in which it is being applied.

FEE-FOR-SERVICE

Perhaps the simplest payment method conceptually because it is how other goods and services are bought and sold in the marketplace, fee-for-service refers to payment for each individual service rendered by a physician to a patient. Prior to the development of medical insurance, physicians defined the services offered, set a price (which might be altered based on the perceived financial situation of the patient), and directly sought payment from the patient. Patients, like any other consumers in the marketplace, retained the option of seeking care elsewhere or going without.

Historically, physicians obviously did better financially by performing services that patients would buy. George Bernard Shaw captured the bias inherent in fee-for-service payment in his preface to *The Doctor's Dilemma* eighty years ago. "That any sane nation, having observed that you could provide for the supply of bread by giving bakers a pecuniary interest in baking for you, should go on to give a surgeon a pecuniary interest in cutting off your leg," he wrote, "is enough to make one despair of political humanity."

The development of private health insurance ratified this particular aspect of American political humanity. Health insurance, which began in the 1930s during the Depression, burgeoned as a result of collective bargaining in the economically expansionary post–World War II years. Under most private insurance and Blue Cross–Blue Shield plans, fee-for-service, with physicians determining the economic value of their own services, became the established method of reimbursement for physician services covered under the benefit structure of most insurance policies.

Nevertheless, third-party payers faced a fundamental problem in adopting a policy of paying the doctor's actual fee. If the patient is largely or totally removed from the financial report impact of the doctor-patient transaction, there is virtually no market discipline: The patient is indifferent to the physician charge and will not question either the price or the necessity for the service provided, at least for services that pose no risk or time commitment. Thus, to moderate payment levels somewhat and to maintain some order in the payment process, insurance companies imposed rules designed to limit their payments at the extreme. Insurance companies generally chose between paying based on a predetermined schedule of allowances, regardless of the charge, or paying up to a limit based on the actual charges of physicians in the geographic area where the service was provided.

Under a fee-schedule approach, patients must pay the difference between third-party payer allowances and doctor fees. If there is too great a discrepancy, patients may feel financial pressure based on their obligations to pay the balance bill, perhaps exerting a dampening effect on physician charges. Under a method that pays based on physician charges, physicians receive a reliably high percentage of their charges and face no impediment to raising fees. It is not surprising, then, that Blue Shield plans, largely controlled by medical societies in the 1950s and 1960s, favored a method of payment called "usual, customary, reasonable" (UCR) that was relatively generous to physicians.

UCR Payment

In a major victory for organized medicine, the UCR payment technique became Medicare's method for compensating physicians when enacted into law in 1965. Translated into the Medicare statute as "customary, prevailing and reasonable" (CPR), the method involves payment for a service limited to the lowest of (1) the physician's billed charge for the service, (2) the physician's customary charge for the service (defined as the physician's median charge for the service during a prior twelve-month period), or (3) the prevailing charge for that service in the community (currently set at the seventy-fifth percentile of all physicians in that community).

Endorsed by Medicare and favored by organized medicine, the UCR approach was adopted by virtually all Blue Shield plans and many indemnity insurers as well; UCR flourished for two decades, to the general benefit of physicians. In the last decade, however, UCR came under attack because of its inherently inflationary incentives.[3] An individual physician has an incentive initially to set high fees and to keep raising them. Where patient cost-sharing is small, the physician has little reason not to keep his or her fees at the upper end of the spectrum of fees in the community. Furthermore, physicians in communities where patients enjoy broad and deep insurance coverage can charge higher fees than can those in communities where patients have to pay a substantial portion of the bill out of pocket.

In addition to its inherently inflationary incentive structure, there are two other major problems with fee-for-service as used by third-party payers. First, distortions are brought about by what private and public payers decide to include in their benefit packages. For example, traditional indemnity insurance often covered tests, procedures, and physician hospital visits, but not patient encounters in the medical office, the most common service provided by the medical profession. In the context of UCR reimbursement, physicians were free to increase the fees for fully covered services to compensate for the fact that patients had to face the charges of the office visits without insurance. Thus, the benefit structures produced a tendency toward internally cross-subsidizing within a medical practice and a bias toward performing tests and procedures.[4, 5]

Second, inherent in any fee-for-service system is the problem of defining the services for which the physician requests payment. Consumers know what a loaf of bread is and how to judge the relative price of that good. Medical services are more mysterious and elusive, certainly to the consumer patient. With increasing complexity and specialization, the American Medical Association assumed responsibility for establishing and updating a coding system that attempts to identify and define all physician services. The common procedural terminology (CPT) was first issued in 1966 and is now in its fourth major edition, with updates annually. Virtually all third-party payers, including Medicare, now recognize CPT as the taxonomy for physician services. The current volume of CPT includes over 7,000 discrete services and still does not accurately describe thousands of variations and permutations in what physicians do and request payment for.

Since the coding scheme is modified every year, with numerous additions, deletions, and redefinitions, it is a moving target for payment purposes. Physicians are able to take advantage of the complexity of the procedural taxonomy and payment rules and the imprecision of some of the code definitions to "creatively" bill, again protected by the fact that the well-insured patient is indifferent to the size and scope of the bill. Examples of creative billing include unbundling (billing separately for activities that have traditionally been considered as part of a single service) and upcoding (billing for a higher level of service than was actually provided). Another form of creative billing is charging the third-party payer for uncovered services, usually preventive health services, by listing false diagnoses.

The complexity and imprecision of the coding system and payment rules virtually invite physician gaming behavior. Indeed, as long as the third-party payer is on the hook, patients in essence conspire with physicians on billing: The more charges that can be shifted to the outside payer, the less out-of-pocket expenditures that they face. Facing a confusing CPT coding system, complicated payment limits, and arbitrary benefit exclusions, physicians have effectively lost control over their own ability to bill patients what they feel their services are worth. In this setting many physicians have few compunctions about getting what they feel they deserve, even though gaming is involved. Physicians vary in how routinely and extensively they attempt to game the insurance-dominated fee-for-service system. While relying on potential criminal sanctions for overt fraud, payers have been unable to effectively combat the ability of doctors to manipulate the fee-for-service system to their own benefit.

To summarize, in unrestricted fee-for-service where the insurer is obligated to pay on behalf of subscribers and has no contractual relationship with physicians, the combination of UCR and CPT results in substantial inflationary pressures on expenditures, with no direct or obvious link to quality of care. Fee schedules are attempts to correct the most inflationary aspects of fee-for-service by limiting the payer's financial liability to levels determined by the fee schedule, rather than by the physician. Alternatively, tighter application of UCR methods can limit liability. For example, by restricting prevailing and reasonable fee increases in a number of ways over the past fifteen years, the Medicare program uses a de facto fee schedule.[6] Nevertheless, a de facto fee schedule based on charges looks different from a designed fee schedule based on resource costs.

Fee Schedules

A primary reason why third-party payers have not moved to applying fee schedules as a means of limiting expenditures is that the fee-schedule allowance may diverge too much from the physician's charge. Where patients remain responsible for paying the difference between the allowance and the doctor's charge, subscribers and beneficiaries may feel shortchanged, especially if they have already incurred substantial premium charges. Indeed, there is often a fundamental conflict between the goals of cost restraint and of patient satisfaction. Or put another way, consumers as subscribers and consumers as patients have different interests.

In situations where physicians by contract can choose whether to "participate" with a particular buyer—for example, Blue Shield plans, Medicare, HMOs, and preferred provider organizations (PPOs)—thereby foregoing the privilege of billing the patient the balance between approved payments and charges, physicians naturally will be less likely to participate where the fee-schedule allowances do not approach expected rates of return on charges. Some physicians may choose to give discounts on their charges, by accepting fee-schedule allowances, in exchange for anticipated increases in patient volume that a participation agreement should bring. Physicians may also be willing to accept reduced fee-for-service payments from a third-party payer because the contractual relationship with the payer is a guarantee of payment, reducing the problem of bad debt from failure to collect from individual patients.

From the payers' viewpoint, a schedule of allowances provides some budget predictability and is easier to administer than a UCR payment system.

The bottom-line question, nevertheless, is whether a fee schedule achieves cost restraint. The simplest fee schedule to put into effect is one that sets the fee limits at some percentage—for example, 75 percent—of area charges for each CPT service. Importantly, applying a fee schedule to a CPT-based physician charge system does not correct the inflationary defects underlying fee-for-service described earlier. Indeed, in participating physician situations where patients are relieved of cost-sharing obligations, as with most HMOs and PPOs, there may be no market discipline at all influencing the fee-for-service incentives. While the individual fees paid according to the fee schedule may be lower than the individual service charges, physicians can generate increases in the volume of services provided—that is, they can "induce patient demand"—at no direct financial cost to the patient. Indeed, HMOs paying fee-for-service anecdotally report an explosion of office visits in recent years.

Even with fee freezes or strictly limited fee increases allowed in recent years, Medicare has nevertheless experienced large annual increases in Part B expenditures, attributed mostly to increases in the volume of services provided and/or billed.[7] Whether the volume increases are justified and result in improved services is a matter of debate.

FEE-FOR-SERVICE REFORM

The focus of attention for Medicare reform of physician payments in recent years has been the resource-based relative-value scale (RBRVS), developed by William Hsiao and his colleagues at the Harvard School of Public Health. The RBRVS has desirable features, especially with regard to promoting greater equity within the profession. However, by itself, there is no reason to expect that a new fee schedule based on the RBRVS will moderate expenditure increases.

In addition, a uniform Medicare fee schedule does not reward quality directly. Under a fee schedule, price is not sensitive to market forces; thus, a higher quality physician cannot benefit by charging higher fees. Some argue that such a system of externally administered fees results in inefficient allocation of health resources with no rewards to efficient or high-quality providers. Nevertheless, a virtue of the fee-for-service, free-access medical system is that doctors compete for the allegiance of patients. Under a fee schedule, high-quality physicians can be rewarded by an increased volume of patients, even if their prices are externally set. This form of resource allocation obviously pertains in areas of physician excess where physicians are not working at capacity.

There are bases for setting fee schedules, other than the inherent resource costs, that might have some cost-control effects.[8] Additionally, paying for bundles of services, as with DRGs, is a payment reform that Medicare adopted for hospital payment. DRGs represent a major coding reform within a context of reimbursement for services. While useful for hospital reimbursement, the applicability of DRGs to physician payment reform is more problematic and not likely, at least in the near term. Other cost-containment options, alone or in combination, include utilization management, practice guidelines, selective contracting, and formal expenditure limits.[4,7] The merits of these approaches must be evaluated in the context of a system in which the predominant incentives are strongly in the direction of increased services. Similarly, most quality assurance activities now focus on eliminating the identified excesses in such a system.

PREPAYMENT

Prepayment turns fee-for-service incentives upside down. Here, a contractually determined, fixed payment, no longer thought of as a reimbursement, is made for a defined set of services, *whether or not the services are actually provided*. The major examples of prepayment in the United States are HMOs, also called prepaid group practices. Here, a subscriber, or an employer on behalf of a subscriber, pays a monthly premium and then faces no out-of-pocket expenses for covered services, except for strictly limited, usually nominal, copayments. Just as the HMO receives a monthly fixed payment and must do business within the budgetary constraints imposed by prepayment, the HMO can turn around and share part of the financial risk with the physicians with whom it contracts.

The open-panel HMO can share its financial risk using fee-for-service payment methods, usually by withholding a percentage of all reimbursements to physicians and then returning part or all of the withheld amounts based on an end-of-year accounting of whether expenditures met budget projections. This form of risk sharing is a form of fee-for-service with an expenditure limit. For the individual physician in the provider network, the incentives remain "more is better."

Capitation

Alternatively, an open-panel HMO can use a more ambitious and fundamentally different technique for placing physicians at financial risk, commonly called capitation. A prototypic capitation program works in the following manner.

A primary care physician (family physician, pediatrician, or general internist, or sometimes gynecologist) contracts with the HMO to provide services to enrollees who select from a list a single physician to be their primary care gatekeeper or case manager. The gatekeeper-physician receives from the HMO a monthly payment by the head (the capitation); this amount is usually adjusted actuarially for each patient's age and sex. The capitation amount, currently about $10 to $12 per head in Washington, D.C., is meant to cover the costs of all primary care services that physicians are obligated by contract to provide, regardless of actual patient utilization. Typically, the HMO retains part of the capitation amount, perhaps 20 percent, as the withhold amount.

For every $10 in capitation, the HMO sets aside another $40 or so in one or two separate accounts to pay for hospital care, specialist physicians care, and ancillary services. The gatekeeper physician must authorize the specialized services that their patients receive, except in emergencies. Annually, the HMO audits the specialized services account. If it shows a surplus, the gatekeeper-physician receives a bonus, as much as 30 to 50 percent of the surplus. If the account shows a deficit, the monthly capitation withholds are drawn down by the HMO. In most situations the physician's financial risk is limited to the amount of withholds. It should be emphasized, however, that there is no limit to the gatekeeper-physician's time commitment to his or her patients under capitation.

Conceptually, the economic incentives of this capitation-risk payment system correct for the abuses of fee-for-service billing described earlier. The incentives are different; under capitation, physicians do better by keeping patients away from consultants and out of the hospital. When these services are needed, they should select lower-priced specialists and facilities that do not require specialized expertise. In theory, the incentives of capitation-risk also promote more vigilant physician behavior, with greater attention to preventive medicine in order to forestall or eliminate avoidable illness that subsequently would deplete referral pools.

In reality, the rationale for the capitation-risk system partly breaks down. The two major problematic issues are actuarial and ethical. There are also a series of accounting decisions, usually made at the discretion of the HMO, that can significantly alter the bottom line for a particular physician.

Actuarial Problems

The first actuarial problem relates to selection bias. When the characteristics of a physician's panel of patients differ systematically from those of the population from whose experience the capitation rates and pool allocations were set, selection bias has occurred. The HMO may have based allocations on national utilization data not particularly relevant to the enrollees in a particular geographic area. Furthermore, age and sex, the additional actuarial measures commonly used to differentiate payment allocations, are very crude predictors of medical care use.

The crude estimates of risk would not be a major problem if, as the payment system assumes, enrollees randomly select primary care gatekeepers. However, different physicians often systematically attract different kinds of patients who present different burdens of illness and needs for medical care. At the present time, models that adjust capitation rates for patient characteristics that influence future utilization, thus minimizing the problem of biased selection, are in a very early stage of development.[9, 10]

A second actuarial problem is that of random statistical variations associated with small numbers. In the model where an individual physician is at risk for his own panel of patients, the adverse experience of a few patients can overwhelm the most cost-effective behavior on routine patient problems. Conversely, a less cost-conscious physician whose case load includes no catastrophic illnesses may do quite well financially. HMOs typically do include stop-loss provisions that limit the amount that can be debited from a physician's pool as a result of a single enrollee's bills. A common stop-loss amount used by HMOs is $5,000. Yet, with a $5,000 stop-loss, a physician who can perform 10 percent better than the budgeted amount on routine patients would have to accumulate 1,000 patient-months of capitation and pool allocations to compensate for the amount lost from just one catastrophic case.

Reduced stop-loss thresholds would partly reduce the actuarial problems associated with small numbers and selection bias. Another approach to the small numbers problem is to group physicians together for accounting purposes. An already existing group practice can be its own pool and can even choose to pay itself its received capitations and bonuses by methods other than capitation.[8] Alternatively, different practices or even all the physicians in an independent practitioner association (IPA) can be grouped. The larger the group, the less often problems arise due to selection bias and variations associated with small numbers. But the larger the group, the smaller the incentives for individual physicians. If the group account is very large, physicians effectively are working for their capitations with little expectation that their personal practice decisions will have any effect on whether they receive a bonus or give back their withholds.

Ethical Concerns

Related to the actuarial problems with capitation-risk is the ethical concern of giving physicians incentives to provide less care. In essence, HMO managers take the same physicians whom they and others criticize for providing unnecessary services in a fee-for-service environment and entrust them not to underserve their captive patients in the face of direct economic incentives to do so. The less care physicians give their patients, the greater the physicians' financial gain. No set of economic rewards and penalties should be necessary to modify physician practice behavior when standard medical practice dictates a course of action. But many medical decisions take place in a gray area. Theoretically, as noted earlier, vigilant behavior is rewarded under capitation because more serious illness that depletes referral accounts can be avoided or forestalled. Unfortunately, truly vigilant care may be a net cost, at least in the short term. Early treatment of hypertension, tight control of blood sugar in a diabetic, recognition of alcohol abuse in functional alcoholics, and nutrition counseling for patients who are obese or have elevated cholesterols may reduce strokes, heart attacks, and accidents that would be likely to occur many years later, long after the patient has moved on to another job, another health plan, and another physician. Furthermore, a great deal of primary care medicine involves quality of life, not life and death or even preventable morbidity. Yet, under the incentives of individual capitation, the primary care gatekeeper has a direct financial incentive to withhold or defer discretionary services related to quality of life.

There is a major countervailing economic pressure on the physician that works to reduce the capitation incentive to withhold necessary or desirable services. If the physician too aggressively shortchanges the HMO's patients, it can complain or transfer its patients' care to others. The physician then loses business or can even be dropped from the HMO. Again, fundamental professional ethics function to preserve the basic doctor-patient relationship. The primary concern is about marginal decisions and whether capitation-risk tilts the balance too far in the other direction from fee-for-service.

SALARY

It is not generally appreciated that many U.S. physicians are compensated for their professional services by salary. Physicians employed by the Department of Defense and the Veterans Administration receive congressionally mandated salaries. Interns and residents are salaried. Most close-panel or group-model HMOs pay their primary care physicians and some specialists primarily on a salaried basis. They may in addition provide relatively small bonuses based on group or individual performance. Finally, many new members of a private group practice may initially be hired on salary. The new physician may generate revenues for the practice on a fee-for-service and/ or capitated basis, but personally receive a salary. Again, any bonus may be based on achieving productivity objectives.

The salaried physician may be somewhat oblivious to incentives that fee-for-service and capitated physicians routinely face because utilization of services is not related directly to compensation levels. What the salaried physician has an incentive to protect is his or her own time, by deferring work or referring patients to others. However, virtually all salaried physicians are in an employer-employee relationship. They have been hired and can usually be fired. Lax work can result in termination or reduced relative salary. The ability of the employer to scrutinize performance and act accordingly depends on factors unique to the organizational and political setting and on the terms of the employment contract. Are doctors unionized? Are they public employees protected by government regulations? Do they have tenure? Does the organization operate in an area of physician excess or scarcity?

From patients' perspectives, receiving care from salaried physicians provides some assurance that the physicians' recommendations for care are not based on their own pocketbook considerations, as they might be under both fee-for-service and capitation arrangements. Correspondingly, physicians practicing on salary are relieved of some of the more unpleasant aspects of calculating the financial impact of clinical decisions.

Salaried physicians may practice in prepayment settings such as HMOs that do attempt to limit services at the margin. Here, in the absence of direct financial incentives on the physician to limit marginal care, there are usually institutional barriers to care—for example, long queues to obtain certain services. Nevertheless, within the limits of the bureaucratic structure established, physicians on salary can remain patient advocates to help them obtain desired services.

NO IDEAL SYSTEM

There is certainly no ideal or correct way to compensate physicians for their professional activities. Fee-for-service helps promote physician autonomy, although, as noted earlier, not as much as originally conceived. In addition, fee-for-service supports a vigorous work ethic among physicians; effort is rewarded. However, fee-for-service is inherently inflationary at a time when cost is becoming a primary consideration for third-party payers and the public at large.

Prepayment, particularly capitation, gives physicians direct rewards for conserving resources to promote cost restraint. Given the current orientation of the health system that more is better, even when it is not, this new reward system may be desirable to provide balance to physician decision making. The problem is that current designs of capitation-risk programs are generally quite crude, ignoring actuarial considerations that affect the fairness of these systems. Perhaps more important are ethical concerns about physicians who might have a conflict of interest under capitation systems. Many physicians can probably function under such systems, perhaps modified, without a serious compromise of their primary agency relationship with their patients, but others may not. In any case, at the very least, patients enrolling in systems that use capitation should do so with their eyes open. Informed of these payment arrangements, many patients would surely join, attracted to cost-control elements of the plan and confident of the professional integrity of the physician they choose as their gatekeeper.

The final payment alternative, salary, is reasonably incentive neutral for the physician. That might help the physician do what is best for the patient, regardless of cost. The concern is that, at least in some settings, salaried practice may promote a lax practice style; there are no direct financial rewards for achieving desired utilization results. Bonuses or salary increases can be used to reward performance if the circumstances permit. For most physicians in private practice, there is no employer and, therefore, no salary option.

As more and more medical care takes place in managed care arrangements—that is, where physicians agree to provide care under contract—physician payment methods will surely evolve. Even today, there are hybrid systems that incorporate elements of fee-for-service, prepayment, and salary. The goal is to figure out how to provide incentives for reducing health spending without seriously compromising quality or patient confidence in the integrity of the medical care system.

NOTES

1. J. Lister, "Special Report: Proposals for Reform of the British National Health Service," *New England Journal of Medicine* 320 (1989): 877–80.

2. K. R. Levit and M. S. Freeland, "DataWatch: National Health Care Spending," *Health Affairs* 7 (1988): 124–36.

3. B. B. Roe, "Sounding Board: The UCR Boondoggle: A Death Knell for Private Practice?" *New England Journal of Medicine* 305 (1981): 41–45.

4. Physician Payment Review Commission, *Annual Report to Congress* (Washington, D.C.: U.S. Government Printing Office, 1988).

5. W. C. Hsiao et al., "Results and Policy Implications of the Resource-Based Relative-Value Study," *New England Journal of Medicine* 319 (1988): 881–88.

6. R. A. Berenson, "Editorial: Physician Payment Reform: Finally," *Annals of Internal Medicine* 107 (1987): 929–31.

7. Physician Payment Review Commission, *Annual Report to Congress* (Washington, D.C.: U.S. Government Printing Office, 1989).

8. J. Hadley and R. A. Berenson, "Seeking the Just Price: Constructing Relative Value Scales and Fee Schedules," *Annals of Internal Medicine* 106 (1987): 461–66.

9. W. McClure, "On the Research Status of Risk-Adjusted Capitation Rates," *Inquiry* 21 (1984): 205–13.

10. J. W. Thomas and R. Lichtenstein, "Including Health Status in Medicare's Adjusted Average per Capita Cost Capitation Formula," *Medical Care* 24 (1986): 259–75.

7

Taming Medical Technology

Richard K. Riegelman

The last few years have been landmark years in the history of medical care. First, we passed the $500 billion mark in annual health care spending, and then we managed to spend more than $2,000 per capita for medical care. Despite the fact that total medical care costs have increased at nearly twice the rate of growth of our gross national product, the income produced by one hour of the average doctor's time has merely kept pace with inflation.[1] However, there are now many more doctors doing more things, and most are ordering more tests and doing more procedures—in other words, using technology. How and why technology is used have become critical issues not only for medical education and the medical profession, but also for society at large. It is now clear that it will be impossible to control the costs of medical care without taming medical technology.

Let us first look at some reasons for the increased reliance on technology and then at three potential strategies for controlling these costs. The reasons technology has increasingly caused medical care costs to rise can be analyzed and recalled by using the mnemonic TUMS, which stands for

Tantilized by Technology
Uncomfortable with Uncertainty
Motivated by Money
Scared by Suit

TANTALIZED BY TECHNOLOGY

Physicians are constantly tantalized by the allure of modern technology. Each new issue of the most respected journals and each new grand rounds by the most acclaimed experts brings to light new ways to evaluate patients. What physician would dare reject the modern miracles that are increasingly part of the practice of medicine? How could any physician help but be impressed with the newest technology-producing images from living patients which remind one of textbook pictures previously available only at surgery or autopsy? Thus, "modern" is the first and often the last word driving the use of technology. What self-respecting hospital could be without a magnetic resonance imager costing in the millions? What self-respecting physician would associate with a practice without the latest in diagnostic and therapeutic technology? The ability to gain access to technology has brought physicians patients, status, and professional self-esteem.

New technologies, like new drugs, are often introduced and paid for in medical practice after their usefulness has been established only for a specific diagnosis or treatment. These indications are part of the formal approval process that the Food and Drug Administration applies to new drugs and more recently to major changes in medical technology. The new technology is often a substantial improvement over existing technology when used for the narrowly defined approved indication. Even if it is expensive, the new technology may be cost effective. That is, the additional expenditure may be worth the additional expense. Once technology is introduced into practice, it is common for physicians to begin to extend the indications and apply the technology to new diagnostic and therapeutic situations. In these new situations the technology may still be useful, but often it no longer represents a major advance. In fact, the new technology is frequently used in addition to rather than as a replacement for the older tests. Thus, many times it merely adds to the expense without adding to the information. In addition, the widespread diffusion of expensive technology has often meant that each institution utilized its equipment only a small percentage of the time.

In an earlier era, many of the advances in medical technology were accompanied and restrained by an element of risk to the patient. Coronary catheterization had the small risk of causing a stroke or myocardial infarction. Liver and kidney biopsy held the risk of bleeding. Thus, despite these techniques' usefulness in specific circumstances, physicians had a reason to be restrained in their use. No such restraint need accompany the newest generation of medical miracles. Magnetic resonance imaging and echocardiography not only can be done without invading the body but also are believed to be free of the dangers attributed to radiation. If they were free of cost, their use could be justified for nearly every patient on every visit. Thus, we are confronted with a new reality. Increasingly, the seductive effects of technology are constrained only by the costs, not by the risk to the patient.

UNCOMFORTABLE WITH UNCERTAINTY

As long as medicine has been practiced, physicians have faced uncertainty. In the old-old days over a decade ago, there was a very easy way to deal with uncertainty: Physicians denied its existence and hid behind the armor of authority. Patients asked no questions, and the pronouncements of the physician were by definition the right ones. Uncertainty was denied and thus eliminated.

Another method of dealing with uncertainty has become the norm in modern American medicine. This approach tries to eliminate uncertainty by testing. Unfortunately, it is a fruitless and dangerous pursuit, but one that American physicians have worked very hard to perfect. Technology is used to minimize uncertainty. Thus, appropriate testing is done to reduce uncertainty; then more testing is done to do even better. Since it is never possible to be certain, it is always possible to justify more testing to reduce the uncertainty a little bit further.

In the not-too-distant past, clinical medicine used the motto "to be complete" to justify ordering many marginal tests. "As long as the patient is in the hospital." "You can never be sure the patient doesn't have X." "If you think of it, order it."[2] These and other similar phrases were and may still be used to justify ordering tests that add little to the diagnostic or therapeutic effort, but plenty to the patient's bill. Ordering "to be complete" is no longer an acceptable approach in an era in which physicians are under increasing social pressure to be efficient.

The desire to utilize technology to reduce the uncertainty of diagnosis, increase the predictability of prognosis, and monitor the outcome of care is a reflex for most physicians. Even when the disease is likely to be self-limiting, physicians have trouble restraining themselves from a definitive diagnosis. When the therapy is the same regardless of the exact diagnosis, physicians still tend to order tests to be sure of the diagnosis, rather than implementing treatment and carefully following up patients.

Physicians increasingly feel the need to use technology to provide evidence supporting their diagnoses. Documentation is often needed for insurance coverage and disability determination, and before the use of surgery or therapies that carry an element of risk. A clinical diagnosis increasingly is a derogatory term, meaning that no tests document the disease, rather than expressing faith in the individual physician's judgment. Thus, physicians often feel the need to test to increase certainty even when there is little to be gained in terms of patient outcome.

It may be difficult for individual physicians to restrain their own use of technology when surrounded by peers and governed by standards of practice that endorse its extensive use. The medical profession itself, however, needs to confront and accept the inevitability of uncertainty. Professional skill and judgment need to be viewed as knowing when and how to tolerate uncertainty.

MOTIVATED BY MONEY

It is not surprising to most Americans to discover that a physician's behavior is affected by economic incentives. Observers of physicians' behavior have found that when physicians are paid for whatever they order, they tend to order more tests, and when given incentives to order less, they tend to respond by restricting their ordering. Some have concluded that physicians' orders can and do create their own demand for services.[3]

Economic forces, however, play a much smaller role in physicians' decision making only when there are well-established professional standards. When clear-cut "official recommendations" are available, physicians who are salaried, capitated, or in fee-for-service practice usually follow these recommendations and order nearly the same tests and prescribe the same therapy. Thus, physicians are most affected by economic incentives when professional recommendations and standards are vague, in conflict, or undefined.[4]

Most American physicians today have a vast array of tests and treatments available at the stroke of a pen. When under time pressure or confronted with a confusing patient or a complex problem, it is tempting to reach for the pen, order the test, and get on to the next patient. Saving time by testing has become a reflex reaction for many physicians who often do not even recognize their own reactions. Financial incentives, to the extent that they play a role, serve to reallocate the use of a physician's time. They often encourage physicians to take the extra time to make the assessment themselves rather than ordering more tests.

SCARED BY SUIT

Malpractice suits occur more frequently and have such financial impact that many physicians regard them as a factor in decision making.[5] There is an additional effect of malpractice on the medical profession which stems largely from physicians' strong desire to protect themselves. Malpractice insurance gives partial financial protection, but physicians still fear suits as though their practice depends on avoiding them. They legitimately fear the dangers to their reputation, the personal emotional turmoil, the attacks on their professional self-respect, and the enormous consumption of their limited time.

Physicians who are scared by suits are tempted to reduce the possibility of error by ordering additional tests to cover all the contingencies. Tests ordered when there is a low probability of a disease can cause more trouble than they are worth. In this situation the probability of a false positive result is high and necessitates further, sometimes dangerous, tests to rule out disease. Thus, the tempting practice of testing to cover all possibilities rarely provides physicians with much protection. Rather, it often makes life more difficult by forcing the physician to decide when enough is enough.

The physician's heavy hand on the pen is often reinforced by patients. Patients have come to equate testing with quality. Those pictures from the scanner or the catheterization are more tangible, more real, and thus more believable than the intellectual synthesis that emerges from the history and physician's examination. A diagnosis without a test no longer meets the patient's expectation.

Physicians often fear they will look bad in court if they fail to make a diagnosis. Fortunately, however, most patients are more sensible. When time is spent explaining the options, most patients will be interested in maximizing the benefits and minimizing the risks of diagnosis. If there is little danger of serious disease, patients are frequently willing to forego the formalities of a definitive diagnosis. Nonetheless, many physicians believe that malpractice protection is an important reason to order what would otherwise be medically unnecessary tests.

WHAT CAN BE DONE?

There are three basic strategies for reducing the total cost of the use of technology. Reliance can be placed on financial incentives, administrative regulations, or professional standards. In all likelihood all three strategies will be needed.

Financial incentives encourage physicians to alter their ordering patterns. Much of the current discussion about options is aimed at finding better payment mechanisms by altering the payment system. The current goal is a payment mechanism in which physicians' ordering is not influenced by financial incentives. Payment reform alone does not ensure that physicians will choose to practice cost-effective medicine. Payment regulation may leave physicians free to order and patients free to pay.

The current stress on a relative-value fee schedule assumes the need to reform the physicians' economic incentives so that their motivations for money can be turned toward making the medical system more efficient. While this may be a worthwhile goal, it cannot by itself hope to completely control costs. Physicians' ordering behavior cannot be controlled exclusively by economic incentives because that behavior is not entirely the result of the motivation to make money.

A second mechanism that can be used may be termed administrative regulation. Administrative regulation in its most extreme form makes certain types of technology unavailable. If an expensive surgery or drug is not approved, it cannot be ordered. If it is available only at a few hospitals or only after prolonged justification, it will not be widely used. This type of administrative regulation removes the decision from the individual physician, and it often removes the decision from the medical profession as well. Administrative regulation ensures reduction of short-term cost, but this may be at the price of reduced quality and increased long-term costs.

There is a third alternative that may be combined with the other strategies, but uniquely requires the active involvement of the medical profession. This third basic strategy is to control the costs of technology based on cost-conscious professional standards. Professional standards are a longstanding part of medical practice. For many years, professional standards were used to elevate the scientific standards of clinical practice. Traditionally, those standards have been developed by specialists in a particular field without regard to cost and often without an appreciation of the consequences of their recommendations when used by the general population of practicing physicians.

When developing professional standards, physicians traditionally have felt an obligation to implement any therapy in which the benefits outweigh the risks, no matter how slightly. No one asked whether the modest benefit was worth the high cost. Physicians, like the Food and Drug Administration, judged the effectiveness of therapy compared to its side effects. Often a risk-benefit analysis suggests use of a treatment without comparing the risk-benefit ratio of one therapy to that of another. Increasingly, we are comparing our treatments. Our comparisons, however, often leave out one important component: the cost of the treatment. Costs have been left to the economists and the administrators. It has been the clinicians' job to advocate for the patient all treatments that have more benefit than risk, no matter how small the benefit.

It is very difficult for physicians to consider costs without sacrificing their role as patient advocates. As individual clinicians, physicians naturally recoil from telling individual patients that the benefits to them are not worth the cost. Even small benefits to the individual patient are often perceived to be worth the cost, especially when these costs are not out-of-pocket to the patient. Recommending against testing or treatment must be done indirectly by setting professional recommendations at a social level. The individual clinician can then implement these recommendations, using these professional standards as indications for or against a therapeutic decision.

There are roles, however, for the individual physician. Individual physicians can help society to avoid the hard decisions by eliminating the use of technologies that have no additional benefit compared to their risks. Physicians can and increasingly are expected to remove the waste from the system, whether that means reducing the length of a hospital stay, ordering only tests that make a difference, or using consultation for advice, rather than transferring the responsibilities for care. Individual clinicians also can contribute to the professional hard work of deciding where to set professional standards. That is, physicians as a profession must be prepared to state that a certain therapy is not cost effective since the extra benefits are not worth the extra cost.

Professional standards provide an alternative and complementary means of taming medical technology. Physicians are very responsive to clear-cut professional standards. When available, these standards often provide a shield for the physician to hide behind, as well as a path for the physician to follow. These recommendations can be incorporated into the Food and Drug Administration's approval process, the recommendations of specialty societies, the textbooks written by experts, and the continuing medical education of medical specialty organizations. The development, dissemination, and attention to official recommendations is now part of the established educational and continuing education process. It is a process that is inherently developed by and for the medical profession, often sanctioned by legal and administrative bodies, and endorsed by insurance payers, both private and governmental. Cost-conscious professional standards may be used to control the costs while retaining most of the benefit.

Professional standards can be used to address each of the four basic reasons for using technology that are incorporated into the mnemonic TUMS. Individual physicians cannot be expected to resist the allure of modern technology on their own. Professionally derived indications that incorporate cost considerations can provide the average physician with a justification for not ordering and a means of restricting those physicians who would stretch the indications.

The desire to be modern may lead to much unproductive ordering or unnecessary therapy. This type of ordering can often be deterred by merely erecting a barrier that requires physicians to justify testing or procedures that go beyond the official indications. Of course, physicians are skillful at fitting the patient to the indications, as well as fitting the indications to the patient. Much of this can be avoided, however, by a randomly selected retrospective peer review of patient care.

Official recommendations can also serve to help physicians deal with the uncertainty inherent in medicine. Official recommendations are often a means of imposing certainty when no such certainty exists. Uncertainty is inherent in the practice of medicine, but the official recommendations usually reflect a consensus outlining what the profession has agreed to do in the face of this uncertainty. Consensus provides a substitute for certainty. It allows the individual physician to feel secure when acting within the consensus and alerts the physician to the need to justify even justifiable deviations from that consensus. Tolerance of uncertainty cannot be legislated or mandated from above. It can, however, be built into official recommendations and professional standards.

When physicians feel the need to do everything possible, they are more likely to order tests to try to eliminate uncertainty. When they are encouraged to do everything proven, as reflected in the official recommendations, they are more likely to hesitate before doing more. Thus, when physicians are given practical, cost-effective professional guidelines, they are likely to stick to the recommendations.

Official recommendations also provide a means to restrain ordering that is motivated by money. This includes the underordering that may also be the result of financial motivation. Even physicians whose primary motivation is financial usually feel the need to justify their orders based on the quality of care or the potential benefits received. Professional standards thus serve as external constraints on the more extreme abuses. The success of this approach, however, requires a formal, ongoing process of monitoring care retrospectively, channeling ordering prospectively, or both.

Finally, professional standards are potential means of controlling the costs of malpractice suits. Those physicians who order unnecessary tests in order to avoid malpractice are probably the same ones who are most likely to adhere to clear-cut official recommendations. This is especially true if these clinicians have a solid basis for believing that such adherence will provide a degree of malpractice protection. Reform of malpractice that strengthens the legal basis for official recommendations may go a long way toward reducing the impact of defensive medicine.

The process of developing professional recommendations and standards is already well underway. Technology assessment and the professional standards that result are now being pursued by individual researchers, medical specialty societies, and a variety of governmental bodies. New players, including the National Institutes of Health and the Institute of Medicine, have given the field increasing respectability and the potential for vastly increased funding. Technology assessment linked with a process of developing official recommendations can go far toward controlling the costs of technology while maintaining most of the benefits. Technology assessment and professional standards will not do the entire job, and they are unlikely to solve all cost problems, but they can help ensure that we receive maximum benefits for the dollars spent.

Technology has become the engine driving both the progress and the costs of medical care. When we talk about the costs of paying the doctor, we must constantly remember that the big bills are what the doctor orders, not what the doctor keeps.

NOTES

1. S. R. Eastaugh, *Medical Economics and Health Finance* (Boston: Auburn House, 1986).

2. J. E. Hardison, "To Be Complete," *New England Journal of Medicine* 300 (1979): 193–94.

3. H. S. Luft, "Variations in Clinical Practice Patterns." *Archives of Internal Medicine* 143 (1983): 1861–62.

4. J. M. Eisenberg, *Doctors' Decisions and the Cost of Medical Care* (Ann Arbor, Mich.: Health Administration Press Perspectives, 1986), pp. 125–38.

5. S. V. Williams, J. M. Eisenberg, L. A. Pascale, and D. S. Katz, "Physicians' Perceptions About Unnecessary Diagnostic Testing," *Inquiry* 19 (1982): 363–70.

8

Competitive Medical Organizations: A View of the Future

John E. Ott

Despite many efforts to contain costs while providing quality care, medical care expenditures continue to rise, and 31 million Americans do not have health insurance. The relative lack of progress in developing cost-effective health care delivery systems suggests that a more radical departure from the current regulatory approach is necessary if there is to be any satisfactory alternative to a national health service in the United States.[1]

The best long-term proactive approach for physicians is to plan, develop, and implement voluntary vertically integrated systems that are payment-neutral competitive medical organizations (CMOs). Voluntary vertically integrated organizations are health care delivery systems in which health care providers affiliate cooperatively and willingly to provide primary, secondary, and tertiary care services in both ambulatory and inpatient settings. Such systems eliminate many of the current problems, such as cost shifting, gatekeeping, and uncoordinated care. CMOs will provide care at the most effective delivery site. Competitive medical organizations, which should evolve over the next few years, are an attractive alternative to national health insurance because they include active participation in the organization by clinicians, foster competition rather than regulation, and lead to cost-effective quality care which will ultimately reduce the rate of insurance premium increases. The emphasis will be on cost-effective care because profits probably will be distributed on the basis of efficient, effective care, rather than by cost shifting from one segment of the system to the other.[2]

Only time will determine whether CMOs of the type to be described here will evolve, but prototype models are already in existence. Inadequate capital and management information systems, as well as the reluctance of physicians to give up some of their professional autonomy for the good of the group,

Figure 8.1
The Competitive Medical Organization

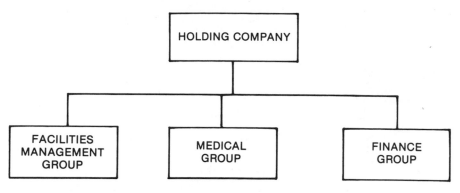

will impede the development of CMOs. However, the alternatives appear even more onerous.

It is doubtful that society will continue to accept the rapidly escalating costs of health care. Our technological abilities already exceed society's willingness or ability to pay enormously increased costs for continued marginal improvements in health care. There appear to be three generic approaches to alleviating this problem. Americans can develop a system rationalizing the rationing of health care on an ethically acceptable basis. A second alternative is the regulatory approach exemplified by a national health service that explicitly rations care by developing eligibility rules, limiting expenditures for health care, establishing fee schedules, etc. Such a system is likely to increase administrative expenses, and health care providers will find methods for evading any rules that are established. Complex as the concept of CMOs is, the concept of competition is probably less threatening to health care practitioners and the public than the other two approaches are, and, therefore, it is likely to be attempted first. If CMOs are unsuccessful, some form of nationalized health service and explicit rationing of care seems likely.[3]

Competitive medical organizations of the type to be discussed do not exist at the present time. Certain elements are seen in existing models, but the total system has not yet evolved. A typical CMO's administrative structure might include four units. The policy-making and decision-making group will be the holding company, which will act for the three remaining groups: the medical, facilities management, and finance units.

The Executive Committee of the holding company might consist of the CEOs of the holding company and of the three subunits and a public representative. The holding company's CEO will probably come from the managed care industry because successful managers in this industry typically are imaginative; have good communication, management, and financial skills; and are used to rapid decision making. The holding company's executive committee will be the governing body that has the authority to contract for the other groups. The five members of the executive committee will have equal votes.

The medical group will be made up of all the clinicians and ancillary staff required to provide medical services, such as primary and specialty physicians; mental health, alcohol, and drug abuse professionals; speech and physical therapists, etc. The medical unit will control the mix of primary and specialty physicians, as well as the number of midlevel practitioners and other health professionals required for the most efficient provider arrangement. Ultimately, participating physicians will probably be operating in a closed-staff network—that is, they will work primarily or exclusively with the CMO.

The facilities management group will be responsible for acquiring, equipping, and maintaining the buildings required to provide care, including hospitals, ambulatory surgery suites, alcohol and drug treatment facilities, medical office buildings, etc. In the future, hospitals will be less important than they are now as more and more care is provided in an ambulatory setting. Routine inpatient care will be provided in community hospitals, while high-technology care logically will be delivered in centralized tertiary care centers that have fewer beds than today's tertiary hospitals.[4] In CMOs, high-technology instrumentation should be centralized because all units will be penalized if cost-effective arrangements are not developed. The finance (venture capital) unit will be responsible for obtaining and managing the financial resources required to achieve the CMO's objectives. The primary sources of funds are likely to be the insurance and pharmaceutical industries which will purchase bonds and seek equity participation in addition to repayment of the loans. One element of participation will be the ability of the insurance and pharmaceutical companies to sell their products at competitive prices to or through the CMOs. The leader of this unit is likely to be chosen from the pharmaceutical rather than the insurance industry. Successful upper-level pharmaceutical managers are the more likely choice because they routinely take significant risks in a world of uncertainty and are better able to make decisions quickly in a rapidly changing environment.

Capital from the finance unit will be used to establish networks or to buy the component parts of the health care delivery system, to develop the extensive management information system required to manage this integrated system, and to coordinate quality assurance, utilization review, and other oversight activities.

The leaders of the CMO will need both an entrepreneurial spirit and the management expertise to run a complex, vertically integrated organization. They are likely to concentrate their activities on improving the quality of care as perceived by both patients and clinicians. Quality of care, as perceived by clinicians, will increasingly consider the clinical outcomes and cost-effectiveness of care. Ethically defensible means of rationing care will have to be developed as society places an absolute limit on the amount of money that will be available to pay for health care. Improving quality of care as perceived by patients will require more attention to problems of access to the system by patients, waiting times, training of personnel, and general patient satisfaction with the care received. Immediate attention will be directed to patient perceptions of quality because they determine whether patients remain in the system. Since it is much more expensive to attract new patients than to retain old ones, it is essential that patient satisfaction issues be carefully addressed. While this is being done, clinicians must also educate patients and employers regarding the importance of clinical indicators of quality of care.[5, 6]

Improved productivity resulting from increasingly improved, cost-effective quality care will be rewarded whether the CMO is a for-profit or nonprofit organization. Any of the component parts of the system might be structured for profit, but the holding company will probably be configured as a nonprofit organization. For-profit components of the system, if purchased, might be offered to their managers on a leveraged buyout basis, which enables the key employees to purchase equity in the company out of its operating profits. This approach would provide incentives for the employees as well as recapitalization and return on investment to the venture capitalists.[7]

Competitive medical organizations will be voluntary, regionally based systems that are linked to a national network. Regional systems can more readily adapt to a rapidly changing local environment, while a national network will be useful in marketing to national accounts and providing out-of-area service to patients. There will be many competitive medical organizations in the United States, but relatively few in any given area. National CMOs will not dominate the industry, but a few networks will be prominent.

The administrative integration of the units will foster interdependence among the groups. The holding company will provide general administration and marketing services and will contract on behalf of all units. The holding company will also be responsible for quality assurance and utilization review throughout the CMO. At present, quality assurance programs evaluate care in the hospital and in HMO ambulatory settings, but rarely do quality assurance programs review episodes of care at all the relevant delivery sites. An episode of care is the element of care provided to a patient with a given problem over time, regardless of the type of professional who provides the care or the setting in which the care is provided. Few organizations know the costs of specific services they are selling, and very few organizations have determined the annual or total costs of episodes of care. Performing these studies through the system will provide realistic data to determine the costs of a particular service.[8, 9]

The CEO of the holding company will negotiate contracts at arm's length with the provider and physical facility components to cover the costs of providing the service and capital required, but will not include profit. Profits will be distributed through the holding company, based on the results of the entire system. Profits might be distributed to the medical, the facilities management, and the financial units in the proportion of 40 percent to 40 percent to 20 percent, respectively. The insurance and pharmaceutical companies would also profit from selling their products. Therefore, each unit would participate in risk sharing which would be tied not only to the financial performance of their component part, but also to the success of the entire organization.

The CMO will have two types of networks. One will be primary care clinics and institutions that will provide referrals for secondary and tertiary care units. The other will be a national network of regional CMOs that will carry out a national marketing program for national corporations and will provide out-of-area coverage for members.

The CMO can provide the personnel, the physical facilities, and the capital to enter into any type of contract, regardless of the payment mechanism utilized. For example, the CMO might provide all the medical specialists necessary to take care of children with complex multisystem congenital birth defects—such as developmental pediatricians, geneticists, orthopedists, plastic surgeons, subspecialty dentists, occupational therapists, and audiologists—in an outpatient multidisciplinary birth defect center. The finance group would provide the capital and fund the hospital that would provide some high-technology secondary and tertiary care facilities as well as the outpatient centers. The facilities management group would be responsible for the operation of the hospital as well as of the ambulatory centers that would house the birth defects center, rehabilitation, genetic counseling, and related medical, dental, and psychological services needed to provide comprehensive care to these children.

What problems can be predicted for competitive medical organizations? There is no organization today that totally fits the description of the CMO. The Kaiser model is as close as any because it combines hospital, medical, and administrative units in related corporations. The component parts of the Kaiser system share resources, but do not share risk with the entire organization. Other systems that include some characteristics of a CMO are the Scripps, Lovelace, and Virginia Mason clinics.

A CMO must be able to make decisions rapidly, something that is very difficult for hospitals, medical centers, and other bureaucratic organizations to do. Because the CMO can provide all services in a one-stop-shopping arrangement, it should be able to negotiate from a strong position. The flexible delivery system can provide a wide variety of benefits and services depending on the specifics of the contract. The integrated management information system and the ability to estimate costs of specific services should make it possible for the CMO to be competitive. Rate setting should be competitive, regardless of the payment mechanism used. The integrated system will permit the CMO's physicians to devote their time to delivering quality care.

Attempts to manipulate the health care system to benefit one of the vested interests will no longer be necessary. There will not be any need to shift costs because all the costs will remain in the organization and the system as a whole will share in the profits. For example, alcohol and drug treatment programs will be carried out primarily in the ambulatory setting since inpatient treatment has not been determined to be more cost effective.

There will be no need for a gatekeeper, so some of the friction between primary care and specialist physicians will be eliminated. If referrals to the specialists are inappropriate, prompt feedback to the primary care physicians should result in behavioral changes. Similarly, specialists will have no incentive to retain referred patients unnecessarily. There will be incentives to provide integrated, cost-effective, multidisciplinary clinics such as cancer centers, diabetic centers, etc., which under prospective payment systems result in adverse selection and severe financial risk to the medical organizations that develop them. Such a multidisciplinary approach might also provide opportunities to contract with insurance companies to care for large numbers of affected patients. For example, an indemnity insurance company could contract to refer large numbers of diabetic patients to a multidisciplinary diabetic clinic. Such a clinic with a well-qualified highly integrated professional staff could provide quality, cost-effective care to the high-risk population. The insurance company could not demand that diabetics receive their care through the CMO, but by providing a financial incentive to the patients through changes in their copayment, deductible, or premium structure, the company could reasonably expect that most of the eligible patients would seek their care at the CMO clinic.[10]

What are the disadvantages that will impede the development of CMOs? The biggest inhibitor is the physicians' need to give up some of their professional autonomy for the good of the group. Physicians are quite independent in their function and have historically typically practiced in solo, private, fee-for-service settings. This trend is eroding, with 50 percent of new graduates of residency programs currently being hired on a salary in group practices. Reduction in individual physician autonomy will be required to obtain the security and the ability to thrive in a rapidly changing external environment. At the same time, individual improvements in productivity must be rewarded. The CMO is capital intensive and will require an elaborate management information system which is not yet available.

Competitive medical organizations will permit physicians to concentrate their efforts on delivering quality care, rather than gaming the system. A vertically integrated CMO will be able to respond rapidly and competitively to any payment scheme that may evolve. This approach should also result in improved care that is responsive to patient needs.

NOTES

1. K. R. Levit and M. S. Freeland, "National Medical Care Spending," *Health Affairs* 7:5 (1988): 124–36.

2. D. M. Berwick, "Health Services Research and Quality of Care," *Medical Care* 27:8 (1989): 763–71.

3. W. Winkenwerder and J. R. Ball, "Transformation of American Health Care: The Role of the Medical Profession," *New England Journal of Medicine* 318:5 (1988): 317–19.

4. G. D. Pillari, "U.S. Hospital Trends in the 1990s: Fewer Beds, Less Debt," *Healthspan* 7 (1990): 13–15.

5. M. D. Merry, "What Is Quality Care? A Model for Measuring Health Care Excellence," *Quarterly Review Bulletin* 13:9 (1987): 298–301.

6. J. W. Williamson, "Future Policy Directions for Quality Assurance: Lessons from the Health Accounting Experience," *Inquiry* 25:1 (1988): 66–77.

7. J. R. Schermerhorn, "Improving Health Care Productivity Through High-Performance Managerial Development," *Health Care Management Review* 12:4 (1987): 49–55.

8. S. M. Shortell, E. M. Morrison, and B. Friedman, *Strategic Choices for America's Hospitals: Managing Change in Turbulent Times* (San Francisco: Jossey-Bass, 1989).

9. S. E. Hartman and D. B. Mukamel, "How Might a Low-Cost Hospital System Look? Lessons from the Rochester Experience," *Medical Care* 27:3 (1989): 234–43.

10. L. L. Roos and S. M. Sharp, "Innovation, Centralization and Growth: Coronary Artery Bypass Graft Surgery in Manitoba," *Medical Care* 27:5 (1989): 441–52.

Part III

Dividing up
the Professions

Pocketbook issues have a way of highlighting special interests. The subject of physician payment can pit professionals against payers at one extreme and specific professional groups against each other at another extreme. Those well-known struggles rarely generate constructive options for the health care needs of society generally. Without ignoring these conflicts, we have also attempted to examine the broad social effect of physician reimbursement issues through the lenses of three sorts of health care provider: the primary care physician, the specialist physician, and the allied health professional.

For Jack Summer, the question is how the primary care physician, viewed as a public resource, can help society attain the widely accepted twin policy goals of reduced health care costs and increased primary care. Of the primary care physician's roles as generalist, preventive care physician, case manager, and gatekeeper, the last puts special pressure on the primary care practitioner. Usual, customary, and reasonable charges or prepayment mechanisms create different variations of these stresses, as does the historically unequal reimbursement rate for primary care. In spite of certain limitations, a resource-based relative-value scale is thus likely to increase the availability of primary care. Summer assesses a number of further innovations that would provide incentives for the increased availability of primary care.

In their survey of specialist reimbursement, Robin Curtis and Robert S. Siegel note that the debate about the privileged role of the specialist began almost as soon as the modern conception of surgical specialization appeared, partly as a result of technical advances during the Civil War. Historically, although physicians have urged government to keep a low profile in the medical marketplace, it was only in the nineteenth century that government got out of the business of regulating prices for health care. Since then, differences in income between specialists and what have come to be known as "cognitively" oriented physicians have provoked sporadic debate, with some groups of primary care physicians recently calling for government to enforce more equity. After a review of some reasons for the spiraling increase in specialist fees, Curtis and Siegel consider the effect of relative-value scales on the availability of specialized services, especially in terms of medical students' career choices.

In some respects the most provocative of the recent and continuing shifts in health care delivery patterns in American society has been the introduction of allied health or "midlevel" professionals, the nurse practitioners (NPs) and physician assistants (PAs). Jean Johnson and James F. Cawley point out that although originally envisioned as supplements for a shortage of physicians, NPs and PAs have become entrenched in their traditional settings such as family practices and outpatient clinics. In a period in which talk of a surplus of providers is increasing, they have also carved out new roles for themselves in specialty practices. These innovations raise questions about payment that go to the heart of the concepts of these relatively new professions, especially with regard to their relationships with physicians and their potential profitability. Perhaps most significantly, the flexibility and affordability of NPs and PAs as providers for certain underserved areas and groups, such as in rural health care and geriatrics, argue for enhanced reimbursement opportunities from public sources.

9

Paying the Primary Care Physician

Jack Summer

For some time, health policymakers have been calling for two significant changes in American health practices: first, the provision of more primary care services, particularly to the medically underserved, with an increase in ambulatory services; and, second, a decrease in health care expenditures which have now reached 11 percent of the GNP and are expanding at a far greater rate than inflation. For example, Medicare spending for physicians increased at an annual rate of 15 percent per year from 1975 to 1987.[1]

To date, very little has been done to reach the first goal, an increase in the provision of primary care services. However, a great deal of effort has been made to accomplish the second, decreased costs. Attempts by government agencies to lower health costs include the initiation of peer review organizations, diagnosis-related groups, and freezes on Medicare and Medicaid physician fee increases. In addition, the private insurance sector is starting to increase the utilization of managed health care systems. One survey made in 1987 revealed that 60 percent of Americans are in some type of managed health care plan.[2] Prepaid health plans have grown rapidly with their own array of cost-saving techniques, including a shift to ambulatory care (with reduced hospitalizations, elective surgery, and medical admissions), risk sharing by participating physicians in independent practitioner associations (IPAs), and stringent utilization review programs. Health maintenance organizations (HMOs) received government's strong initial financial and regulatory support through the 1973 Health Maintenance Organization Act and have continued support today through the growing number of prepaid Medicare and Medicaid contracts which are considered to be partial solution to high government health care expenditures. Prepaid programs (HMOs, IPAs, etc.) are predicted to account for up to 44 percent of all insured Americans by the year 2000.[3]

The twin health policy goals of reduced costs and increased primary care services can be achieved through the increased use of primary care physicians and through more equitable reimbursement to primary care physicians.

ROLES OF THE PRIMARY CARE PHYSICIAN

The place of the primary care physician (PCP) in the health care field today has taken on new importance and complexity because of the trend toward managed health care. The new roles that PCPs must play require management skills and knowledge not traditionally taught or emphasized in our health education system. In addition, many skills and procedures required by these new roles are either inadequately reimbursed or not reimbursed at all in our present physician fee system. Broadly, the PCP plays at least four roles.

1. *Generalist.* The great majority of PCPs are specialty trained, with many programs now developed to specifically train primary care internists and pediatricians. Fellowship programs in ambulatory medicine are beginning to flourish and are necessary to fully train physicians in the wide scope of knowledge and skills required of a properly trained generalist. Family practice residencies have also increased, and the specialty of family practice has gained acceptance; yet board-certified family practitioners are often reimbursed at a level similar to that of general practitioners who have only one year of postgraduate training.[4] The cost-effectiveness of one physician's being able to properly evaluate and manage the numerous problems of an individual or a family seems not to be in doubt. A PCP could reduce the volume of services brought on by multiple specialty visits and, at the same time, increase the efficiency, safety, and convenience of medical care to the patient. The greatly expanding role of the PCP in the evaluation and management of the HIV-positive population is a fitting example. The PCP is starting to assume responsibility for all aspects of care, rather than referring HIV patients to multiple specialists.

2. *Preventive Medicine.* As Americans have become more health conscious, greater emphasis has been placed on preventive medicine, which predominantly falls to the PCP. Whether it is counseling on alcohol, drugs, or AIDS, or screening for cancer or cardiac risk factors, or updating immunizations, much of a PCP's time and effort goes into these endeavors. Traditionally, health insurers pay little or nothing for these services, despite the benefit of these services in reducing rates of infectious, cardiac, and some cancerous diseases. By insisting on high out-of-pocket payments, insurers discourage the public from seeking these highly effective and safe services. If health insurance paid for these services, there could be a rise in the volume of these services and a further step toward reaching the goal of a healthier

society. While an increase in the volume of preventive or health maintenance services would cause an initial increase in cost, the benefits of early health intervention through immunizing, counseling, and evaluating the population for nutritional, cardiac, and cancer risk factors—as well as looking at adverse health behaviors (i.e., drugs and alcohol, smoking, high-risk sexual behavior)—must ultimately lead to reduced costs from disability, morbidity, and premature mortality. For example, the provision of more adequate prenatal care services to women who are at high risk of delivering a low-birthweight infant could reduce total expenditures for direct medical care of their low-birthweight infants by $3.38 for each additional $1.00 spent on their prenatal care.[5]

3. *Case Manager.* In this age of specialization and technology, the PCP spends a significant amount of time coordinating and explaining the health care given, while trying to reduce marginal, harmful, or redundant services. As the physician who knows the patient and his or her needs best, the PCP's role is to help decide which specialist, procedures, or tests are most appropriate. The PCP must assemble all the data (often from numerous sources) to properly manage the patient. The amount of time needed to coordinate care, but not used directly to evaluate or manage the patient, is again poorly reimbursed. It is this activity that is often the most frustrating and stressful to the physician and important to the patient.

4. *Gatekeeper.* With the advent of prepaid and managed health systems, the role of the PCP not only as the case manager, but also as the approver of insurance payments for medical services has evolved. Increasingly, the PCP is being asked to play the role of insurance agent in deciding whether payment for a particular service is indicated. At the same time, the PCP must continue in the traditional role of patient advocate. The decisions are often difficult, especially when determining whether services are medically necessary, medically elective, or marginal, a fine point on which the decision of payment is sometimes based. Not a day goes by that the PCP does not order specialty consultations, hospitalizations, invasive procedures, or laboratory and radiologic evaluations. Now, the physician as well as the patient may have to bear direct financial responsibility if, for insurance purposes, the medical service is deemed excessive or unnecessary. This is a new role that has emerged over the last decade, one for which there is little or no training. This role entails significant stress, especially because it may undermine the doctor-patient relationship and has the potential for causing legal liability. When the insurance company is also the PCP's employer, as in a staff-model HMO, the PCP feels indirect and sometimes overt pressure to care for patients in a manner not compatible with traditional practice styles. The conflict of interest inherent in being a patient advocate and an agent for the insurance company demands that PCPs re-evaluate their practice styles for cost-effectiveness without jeopardizing patient care or comfort. This is certainly possible, but is a specialty in its own right and requires

constant vigilance on the part of the clinician to ensure the interest of the patient is best served.

ETHICAL DILEMMAS OF THE GATEKEEPER

The ethical considerations of the gatekeeper role have been considered by others[6] and bring additional complexity to medical practice. Traditionally, physicians have profited by ordering the marginal, low-risk, low-yield test in a traditional fee-for-service practice with no incentive to be cost conscious. Yet there is no proof that "more" is necessarily "better" medicine. This practice style has been accepted because of our society's attitude of leaving no stone unturned in the search for perfect health care. The new scenario of prepaid medicine is that the physician may profit by not ordering the marginal test or service. The physician may profit financially by reducing health costs as a participant in a bonus system in a staff-model HMO or IPA or as a stock owner in a for-profit HMO. The physician's role now is to show that "less" is not "worse" medicine. The physician in a traditional fee-for-service practice with a small proportion of prepaid patients must also fight the temptation of following two distinct standards of care. Despite the PCPs being the key to cost-effective medicine, again there is no acknowledgment or reimbursement for this role, which is increasingly stressful and requires training and expertise in the medical and ethical complexities of effective gatekeeping.

FINANCIAL DISINCENTIVES FOR PCPs

The present reimbursement system encourages urban or suburban as opposed to rural or inner city practices, as well as specialty- and hospital-oriented practices as opposed to primary care–oriented practices. These factors work against achievement of the goals mentioned previously. The Physician Payment Review Commission's 1988 report to Congress states that the current reimbursement system is creating patterns of allowed charges that embody inappropriate incentives for use of medical services as well as physician decisions on where to locate and what to specialize in.[7]

The present system of "usual, customary, and reasonable" (UCR) payment is regarded by many as flawed because it assumes a perfect marketplace with complete freedom of choice on the part of patients and physicians. There is very reasonable concern that, in fact, the UCR system operates in an imperfect marketplace and that it has distorted physician charges. The market is not truly competitive because of, first, the extensive, but uneven use of health insurance and, second, the fact that sick patients have difficulty acting as rational consumers. These factors have reduced the public's sensitivity to medical fees. Therefore, the public is willing to pay (or have insurance pay) almost any price, and, thus, market forces have not driven prices down to marginal costs.[8] The exception to this is in the area of primary care preventive services where insurance traditionally pays minimally or not at all. An argument can be made that many primary care service fees alone have been carved out of the traditional insurance reimbursement system and have become much more competitive in price because insurance has not masked the true cost of preventive services. Demand for these services is proportionally lower because of higher out-of-pocket expense, and this has driven fees lower than in other areas of medicine. Thus, financial disincentives have been established that discourage physicians from entering primary care fields and practicing preventive medicine in general.

The other end of the spectrum shows that the infatuation of the public, as well as of the medical system, with high technology has lead to an initial overinflation of fees for technology. Unfortunately, as the technology becomes routine and costs are reduced, fees are hardly ever adjusted downward. This encourages fee inflation for procedure-oriented services and incentives for physicians to choose technology-based practices. Again, this implies more urban, hospital-based practices. The present marketplace reimbursement system of UCR payment reinforces trends not desirable for making clinical decisions, choosing specialization, or deciding practice locales.[9] The current reimbursement system undoubtedly has a strong influence on medical graduates and their practice choices.

THE EFFECT OF REASONABLE PCP FEES ON VOLUME AND COST

Physician payment not only has a direct effect on health care costs, but also, by influencing physician behavior, may have a far greater indirect impact on total health care expenditures by affecting the volume of medical services. An analysis by the Physician Payment Review Commission in its report to Congress in 1988 attributes 42 percent of Medicare's increased expenditures to price increases, 44 percent to an increase in the volume of services, and only 14 percent to increased enrollment.[10] Physicians may directly influence up to 70 to 80 percent of all health care spending.[11] As the present fee schedule has underpaid cognitive and primary care services relative to surgical and diagnostic procedures, the incentive has been to increase the volume of services, especially technological tests and procedures. Even the PCP has more incentive to perform office-based diagnostic tests to compensate for fees that favor procedure-oriented physicians. Financial, rather than clinical, factors may lead to some unnecessary services, especially those diagnostic tests perceived as profitable. This coincides with a rise of physician-owned diagnostic centers where the ordering physician gains financially from an increased volume of diagnostic tests.

An analysis of the Medicare fee freeze from 1984 to 1986 revealed a 29.5 percent increase in payment for physician services, two thirds of which were for services that are physician-initiated, rather than patient-initiated, such as surgical, radiologic, and diagnostic procedures. Although a number of events contributed to this rise, "[a]n increase in volume in response to the fee freeze is a real possibility."[12] The ideal market fails here because the patient must rely on the physician not only as the supplier of services, but also often as the sole source of information on which to base decisions about treatment. Price usually plays very little role in the patient's decision because insurance pays for the great majority of these services. Therefore, it can be argued that fees have a direct impact on the volume and intensity of services because physicians adjust the number of tests and visits to maintain their income.[13] Improved payment for cognitive, nonprocedure-oriented services could reduce the incentive for marginal testing, thus possibly reducing total health care costs.

THE RESOURCE-BASED RELATIVE-VALUE SCALE AND ITS EFFECT

The PCP's concern about unequal reimbursement and reduced income compared to other specialties has intensified recently because the trend is worsening. PCPs in general are continuing to lose net real income, compared to their associates. The average physician in 1986 earned $119,500 and the average surgeon $162,400. Yet broken down, in net real income, from 1975 to 1986 anesthesiologists' income rose 2.6 percent per year, surgeons' rose 1.8 percent per year, and radiologists' rose 1.2 percent per year, but internists' fell 0.4 percent per year, pediatricians' fell 0.6 percent per year, and family and general practitioners' fell 1.1 percent per year.[14]

William Hsiao and his associates at Harvard University published the results of their work on the resource-based relative-value scale (RBRVS) in September 1988.[15] This study clearly showed what had been suspected for some time. There is overpayment for surgical and diagnostic procedures relative to evaluation and management services. The study's conclusion, based on evaluation of physician work intensity and time, practice costs, and the opportunity costs for medical education, was that fees for invasive procedures should be reduced by an average of 42 percent and fees for evaluation and management services increased by 56 percent. Specifically, on the extreme end of the scale, the payments to such technology-oriented specialties as ophthalmology and thoracic surgery would be reduced by 40 to 50 percent, and the payments to evaluation- and management-oriented specialties such as family practice would increase by 60 to 70 percent. This was the largest and most accepted study confirming how greatly our traditional UCR fee schedule has deviated from payment based on physicians' resource costs. It showed current, clear inequities of payment when calculations of physician time and effort and other "costs" are considered.

The RBRVS has certain limitations because it is based solely on physician costs. Although correct in assuming that current reimbursements are inaccurate because of the adverse effect health insurance has on a competitive market, the RBRVS has problems in other areas. It does not account at all for patient demand, and price should reflect at least to some degree what the patient's perception is of the worth of the service. Our technology-oriented society may be willing to pay more for surgical and diagnostic procedures; yet, with growing awareness of the need for prevention and health maintenance, individual and social demand could increase the price for primary care services. The RBRVS does not incorporate treatment outcome or the social benefits of a service in its scale, nor does it incorporate the competency of the physician or the quality of the services performed. Finally, there is no consideration in the RBRVS of the variations of patient mix among similar types of practice.[16] Given our present fee schedule, it should come as no surprise that some overpriced procedures have been inappropriately overutilized despite the lack of proven efficacy for improving patients' long-term outcomes. Such procedures as permanent pacemakers, cardiac catheterization, upper GI endoscopy, and carotid endarterectomy have come under scrutiny.[17]

The implementation of the RBRVS will result in a redistribution of payment by specialty, with PCPs being paid more for their predominantly evaluation and management services, and surgical- and procedure-oriented specialties being paid less. In addition, there are other potential benefits. Practice patterns may change toward less surgery and hospitalization and more ambulatory visits. Ultimately, there may be a shift toward an increased offering of primary care services. Consequently, total health care costs may decrease even if the total payment to all physicians remains budget neutral.

INCREASING PRIMARY CARE SERVICES TO THE MEDICALLY UNDERSERVED

A major concern with the health care delivery system is the unequal distribution of physician manpower, resulting in large numbers of medically underserved Americans, predominantly in rural and inner city settings. The RBRVS system does have a geographic conversion factor to establish a fee schedule in each locality. The HCFA's preliminary indications are that there will be a major redistribution of payments between urban and rural areas. This redistribution reflects the increased payments for primary care services that are more predominant in rural areas and the reduced payments to specialty- and procedure-oriented services more commonly found in urban areas. Thus, some direct benefit to underserved areas may occur by way of better reimbursement to many physicians in these areas. The greater part of the effect the RBRVS will have on underserved areas will probably be indirect. If there is relatively less financial incentive to be subspecialty trained or hospital oriented, and relatively more incentive to be primary-care trained, a larger trickle-down effect may be seen in physician shortage areas. Although helpful, more will almost certainly be needed to attract physicians to these areas. An incentive system is beyond the purpose of the RBRVS, but could be a goal of health policymakers and the legislature.

To further improve services to physician shortage areas, the RBRVS's geographic conversion factor could purposely be weighted higher for defined underserved areas, rather than just accounting for "relative work." An argument can be made that the opportunity costs to a physician would be higher, based on the actual or perceived sacrifices an individual makes personally and professionally to practice in a shortage area. This could justify a higher conversion factor for geographically underserved areas and improve the financial attractiveness of practicing in these areas.

Other financial incentives for encouraging medical services to the underserved include reinstituting the Public Health Service Medical School Loan Program, particularly as medical school tuition is escalating and graduates are burdened with tremendous debt early in their careers. High debt may influence young physicians to seek lucrative specialties as a financial necessity.

It makes financial sense to encourage PCPs to practice in underserved areas as a cost-effectiveness measure as well as a measure to help society in general. Medical services in these areas are very costly. For example, inner city emergency rooms with their high overhead, lack of continuity, and poor preventive services are often filling the gap for ambulatory primary care services. Studies of preventive health services to the poor and underserved in other areas have shown that the initial monetary investment has more than been made up in reduced total health care costs.[5] Financial incentives for primary care services may well "pay off" in the same way.

It is unfortunate that arguments about paying the PCP seem based on the relative worth of various services and procedures and thus pit one specialty group against another. The battle line is forming with endorsement of the RBRVS coming from such groups as the American Society of Internal Medicine and skepticism about the plan coming from surgeons. Medical practice has never been homogeneous, and tensions among practitioners are inevitable as government, employers, and third-party payers initiate much more aggressive and restrictive reimbursement systems. Greater competition for patients is a reality as well. According to the Graduate Medical Education National Advisory Committee, in 1970 there were 156 physicians per 100,000 people. By 1980 this had changed to 197/100,000, and the projections are for 260/100,000 by the year 2000. Some have calculated that HMOs require 120 physicians/100,000, and if 44 percent penetration of the market by HMOs is realized by the year 2000, that could increase to 500,000 physicians for 150 million fee-for-service patients or 330/ 100,000.[18] There is little doubt that financial considerations must affect the quality and type of services performed by both PCPs and other specialists, especially as the health care expenditure pie is seen as shrinking.

RATIONALES FOR BETTER PRIMARY CARE REIMBURSEMENT

A number of arguments have been made for increasing the fee-schedule and reimbursement rates to PCPs.

1. PCPs are playing a much more complex role today. They need more training in their expanding role as generalists. Also, they need training to enhance their skills as case managers and gatekeepers in order to effectively balance the often conflicting interests of patients, insurance companies, and traditional practice patterns. Over the last decade, the time and effort required for PCPs to evaluate and manage cases have increased considerably.

The RBRVS is one of the first systems that acknowledges and attempts to correct the present reimbursement inequities. Other systems and refinements will undoubtedly appear that will take into account some of the problems inherent in the RBRVS, but it is clear the "relative value" of primary care services is finally being put into its proper perspective.

2. Increased payment to the PCP may, in fact, help reduce total health care costs by indirectly reducing the number of marginal or unnecessary procedures performed and by helping to reduce the volume of services. The decreased volume of services may occur because there is less financial motivation to supplement income with additional visits or more lucrative procedures.

3. The most important benefit of increased payment to the PCP may lie in its changing health care priorities. Without the financial disincentives now in place, a shift toward more primary care services, especially in underserviced rural and inner city areas, may become apparent. Presently, primary care is often viewed in medical schools as unexciting and unrewarding. The true value of primary care services to the community and society in general is often lost to the medical student, other health professionals, and the public. Financial reimbursement gives very clear signals of worth and esteem. An upgrading of the PCP's image, with increased or at least more equitable financial reward, will be necessary before we are able to give medical graduates the proper signals and truly approach our goal of increased primary care services, especially to the medically underserved.[19]

NOTES

1. W. Roper, "The Resource-Based Relative Value Scale," *Journal of the American Medical Association* 260 (1988): 244–46.

2. J. Gabel et al., "The Changing World of Group Health Insurance," *Health Affairs* 7:3 (Summer 1988): 48–65.

3. Physician Payment Review Commission, *Annual Report to Congress* (Washington, D.C.: U.S. Government Printing Office, 1988).

4. Ibid., 85.

5. Committee to Study the Prevention of Low Birthweight, *Preventing Low Birthweight* (Washington, D.C.: National Academy Press, 1985).

6. G. Povar and J. D. Moreno, "Hippocrates and the Health Maintenance Organization," *Annals of Internal Medicine* 109 (1988): 419–24.

7. Physician Payment Review Commission, *Annual Report to Congress* (Washington, D.C.: U.S. Government Printing Office, 1988), p. 39.

8. P. Ginsburg, "Physician Payment Policy in the 101st Congress," *Health Affairs* 8:1 (Spring 1989): 5–20.

9. W. C. Hsiao, "RBRVS" (Speech presented at the 116th Annual Meeting of the American Public Health Association, Boston, November 1988).

10. Physician Payment Review Commission, *Annual Report*, 1987.

11. George Washington University National Health Policy Forum, *The Proliferation of Physician Services*, Issue Brief no. 508 (Washington, D.C.: January 1989).

12. J. B. Mitchell, G. Wedig, and J. Crumwell, "The Medicare Physician Fee Freeze, What Really Happened?" *Health Affairs* 8:1 (Spring 1989): 31.

13. For a review of the subject, see J. R. Gabel and P. Rice, "Reducing Public Health Expenditures for Physician Services: The Price of Paying Less," *Journal of Health Politics, Policy and Law* 9:4 (Winter 1985): 595–609.

14. Physician Payment Review Commission, *Annual Report*, 1988, p. 34.

15. W. C. Hsiao et al., "Results, Potential Effects, and Implementation Issues," *Journal of the American Medical Association* 260 (1988): 2429–35.

16. W. C. Hsiao, "RBRVS."

17. M. C. Chassin et al., "Does Inappropriate Use Explain Geographic Variations in the Use of Health Care Services," *Journal of the American Medical Association* 258 (1987): 2533–37.

18. Physician Payment Review Commission, *Annual Report*, 1988, p. 32.

19. The Physician Payment Review Commission's report to Congress in 1989 endorsed with slight modification the RBRVS proposal by Hsiao and his associates. This has resulted in a provision in the 1989 Omnibus Budget Reconciliation Act (P. L. 101–239) for an RBRVS to be implemented beginning January 1, 1992, and phased in over five years for Medicare payments. This plan will gradually increase payments to primary care physicians and reduce payments to surgical specialties.

10

Reimbursement and the Specialist: A Historical Perspective

Robin Curtis and Robert S. Siegel

The evolution of medical and surgical subspecialties over the last one hundred years has triggered an ongoing debate regarding appropriate fee structures. At a time of rising medical school tuition and decreasing government support for medical training and payment for medical services, such questions have assumed greater importance as all groups attempt to protect current payment levels. In this chapter, pertinent subspecialty reimbursement issues are discussed, following a brief historical overview of the development of medical and surgical specialties and subspecialties.

SPECIALIZATION IN AMERICA

Dominated by both physicians and laymen, colonial American medical practice differed radically from the more formalized British guild system. Most early American students were educated through apprenticeships, their training limited by the scope of their teachers' mastery of early medical science (p. 149).[1] At a time when illness and personality defects were regularly attributed to imbalances of "the humours" (p. 38),[2] most early American physicians were general practitioners.

Specialties began to emerge in the 1860s when researchers recognized that no universal explanation of all illness is possible in a human body containing multiple organ systems (p. 17).[3] Dramatic advances such as the development of anesthesia, new sanitary techniques, and technological improvements resulting from the study of Civil War casualties heralded a new era of American medical practice, the age of the surgical specialist (p. 24).[3]

The controversy that accompanied development of specialties can be il-

lustrated by this summary of an American Medical Association (AMA)
meeting held in 1866:

This year was notable for the majority and minority reports of the Committee on
Medical Ethics dealing with specialization. The majority report listed the advantages
of specialization as minuteness in observation, acuteness in study, wideness of observation, skill in diagnosis, multiplicity of invention and superior skill in manip-
ulation. The disadvantages were a narrowness of view, a tendency to magnify unduly
the diseases which the specialty covers, a tendency to undervalue the treatment of
special diseases by general practitioners, some temptation to the employment of
undue measures for gaining a popular reputation and a tendency to increased fees.
The advantages far outweighed the disadvantages from the point of view of the
patient and of the advancement of the specialty. The committee felt that these
disadvantages could be overcome if the specialist would begin as a general practitioner and gradually grow into his specialty. (p. 17)[3]

Although most surgical procedures were restricted to trauma cases prior
to the advent of anesthesia in 1846, most subsequent specialty advances
involved surgery. As surgery became more complex, surgeons attempted to
prevent general practitioners and less skilled surgeons from engaging in
surgical practice. General practitioners soon perceived the emergence of
specialties as an encroachment on their domain of practice and as a threat
to their credibility as physicians (p. 24).[3]

The exclusion of general practitioners from several large urban hospitals
precipitated the organization of the American Academy of General Practice
in 1947. Twenty-two years later, general practice, renamed family medicine,
achieved recognition as a medical specialty (p. 19).[3]

THE CONTEMPORARY DEBATE

Over one hundred years after the AMA addressed the controversial development of specialized medicine, the question whether physicians are fairly
compensated for their treatment of patients continues to evoke debate.
Primary care physicians maintain that specialists have a "tendency to increased fees,"[3] just as they did in 1866. In an editorial calling for "adequate
reimbursement of primary care as well as for procedures,"[4] Daniel J.
McCarty laments the results of the 1987 National Residency Matching
Program (NRMP). According to McCarty's interpretation, an increasing
number of America's top medical school graduates are forsaking the cognitive primary care specialties (i.e., internal medicine, family practice, and
pediatrics) so that they may pursue careers in the technology-oriented subspecialties of surgery and the specialties of orthopedics, ophthalmology,
anesthesiology, and radiology. Charging that the primary care physician
must endure greater emotional involvement with patients, more arduous
working conditions, and less predictable hours than procedurally oriented

specialists, McCarty wrote that "the chief reason for its decline in favor with students is that internal medicine continues to be a demanding field that is not nearly as economically rewarding as some others" (p. 569).[4]

According to the 1987 *Medical Economics* Continuing Survey of office-based physicians, this view appears well founded. Of thirteen specialties surveyed, primary care physicians (i.e., internists, family practitioners, pediatricians, and general practitioners) earned $72,840, the lowest median net physician incomes in 1986.[5]

By contrast, surgical subspecialists earned the highest incomes, and neurosurgeons enjoyed the highest median net income, $203,570. Summarizing the survey's results, Arthur Owens writes that "[i]n general, surgical specialists netted more than twice as much as GPs, 69 percent more than FPs, and 38 percent more than non-surgical specialists, even though primary care doctors far outpaced their surgical colleagues in the rate at which their income grew last year" (p. 219).[5]

Kirchner also found that the greatest percentage increase in fees was recorded by primary care physicians. In one attempt to explain this pattern, Lawrence Morris, senior vice-president for health benefits management of the Blue Cross and Blue Shield Association, suggested that the complex case mix of primary care physicians may justify this increase in fees, but that the rate of increase could pose a problem.[6]

Historically, physicians have supported federal legislation in health care matters only when it did not affect their control of the medical marketplace. Although the Virginia House of Burgesses established a fee schedule for physicians' services in 1736, the role of the state in the determination of fees subsequently diminished, especially in the latter years of the nineteenth century. In recognition of the Virginia fee schedule and the passage of laws in Massachusetts (1633) and Virginia (1669) stipulating that physicians charging exorbitant fees were subject to punishment, Paul Starr noted that "before the rise of laissez faire ideology in the nineteenth century, government played an active, explicit, and direct role in economic life that included the regulation of prices" (p. 62).[2]

However, in recent years, the American Society of Internal Medicine (ASIM) has offered legislative support for what it views as a more appropriate fee schedule for cognitive services. In 1980 the ASIM defined cognitive services as "the comprehensive and humanistic application, based upon broadly relevant medical knowledge and experience, of such skills as data gathering and analysis, planning, management, problem solving, decision making, judgment and communication of health problems to the patient" (p. 1).[7] Since that time, ASIM's members have testified before various congressional committees to promote the cognitive services concept.

The issue of physician reimbursement is being debated at a time when Congress is making attempts to reform the Medicare system as a whole. Prior to 1970 escalating medical care costs were considered to be the problems of individuals and their families. Starr suggests that public officials confronted with rapidly increasing national health expenditures, up from $142 to $336 per capital between 1960 and 1970, "began to regard the aggregate costs of health care as too high and to doubt that the investment was worth the return in health" (p. 384).[2] Starr also observes that faulty financial arrangements enabled and encouraged hospitals and physicians to boost their fees (p. 384).[2] An analysis of Medicare's development reveals that the faults of the system may be traced to the emergence of health insurance in this country.

THE ROLE OF HEALTH INSURANCE

In 1929 over 1,200 Dallas, Texas, schoolteachers agreed to pay Baylor University Hospital an annual premium of $6 in return for the provision of a maximum of twenty-one days of semiprivate hospitalization per year. The agreement was the precursor of the eighty-two autonomous Blue Cross plans which provided hospitalization insurance for over one-third of the U.S. population in 1987.

Ten years later, in 1939, a group of California physicians established the first of the Blue Shield plans to insure physicians' services (p. 28).[1] In contrast to Blue Cross managers, who have always insisted that the plans were "community-sponsored effort[s] and democratically controlled," the Blue Shield planners freely admitted their personal interest in the plans' success, claiming that the medical profession has a right to protect its economic interests (p. 308).[2] Blue Shield was designed, in part, to help prevent the implementation of a compulsory federal insurance plan. Many doctors feared that "any financial intermediary [which would accompany such a government plan] would ultimately impose controls on their incomes" (p. 299).[2]

When laying the foundation for Medicare in the early and mid-1960s, Congress and the Johnson administration were eager to win the support of both physicians and hospitals. Consequently, Medicare legislation allowed hospitals to name organizations that could act as fiscal intermediaries between the hospitals and the Social Security Administration. While most hospitals nominated Blue Cross as the agency to provide reimbursements, consultations, and audits, Blue Shield plans assumed similar roles, acting as intermediaries for physicians. When assessing the direct relationship between Medicare and the "Blues" as one of the main structural faults of the Medicare system, Starr writes that "the administration of Medicare was lodged in the private insurance systems originally established to suit provider interests. And the federal government surrendered direct control of the program and its costs" (p. 375).[2]

Rather than reimbursing physicians according to a fixed fee schedule, Medicare adopted the "usual, customary, and reasonable" (UCR) system of reimbursement, which was in the initial stages of development by several Blue Shield plans at the time of Medicare's legislative passage in 1965.[8] Today, Blue Shield plans maintain independent Medicare and private reimbursement profiles.

Over the years, the UCR system of reimbursement has encouraged exploitation. Physicians, claiming they had no record of "usual, customary" fees, charged unprecedented amounts for their services and were paid in full. When other physicians then raised their fees to comparable levels, the "customary" fee increased (p. 385).[2] In this fashion, medical fees and Medicare costs skyrocketed. Starr believes that the lack of effective cost restraints is neither coincidence nor legislative oversight:

It is . . . the outcome of a long history of accommodation to private physicians, as well as to hospitals and insurance companies, which in their own internal organization had adjusted to the practitioners' interests. This institutional phalanx succeeded in blocking any form of control or any alternative form of organization that would have threatened their domination of the market. (p. 387)[2]

Evidence of such domination was documented by a 1979 study of Blue Shield plans. At that time the governing boards of thirty-one out of sixty-nine plans contained a majority of physicians. The D.C. Blue Shield governing board then consisted of twenty-five voting members, twenty-three of whom were elected by participating area physicians. Of those twenty-three, thirteen were required to be physicians nominated by local medical societies. Ten of the practicing physicians serving on the D.C. Blue Shield board in 1979 were surgical or procedure-oriented specialists. The remaining four were primary care physicians. Despite their insistence that they knew "of no instances in which membership on a Blue Shield board or committee led a given physician to benefit directly from actions taken as a member," Thomas Delbanco, Katherine Meyers, and Elliot Sengal emphasized that primary care physicians should be more equitably represented as Blue Shield trustees:

The data from D.C. Blue Shield and several other plans indicate that procedure-oriented specialists predominate, particularly on committees relating directly to fees. A shift to more equal representation might stir debate among physicians and provide a means within the profession to correct imbalances. (p. 1319)[9]

L. Gregory Pawlson attributes the discrepancies existing among physician fee schedules to the combined effects of the UCR mechanism of reimbursement and the implementation of Medicare itself.[10] According to Pawlson, a direct correlation exists between the development of new medical services and the increased medical costs. In a typical market the cost of a new service decreases as usage becomes more common or as a commodity becomes easier to produce. In this respect the medical market deviates from normal economic behavior. When a fee for a new procedure is set, the fee is rarely reduced as the procedure becomes more common and less difficult to perform. To date, physicians have never voluntarily reduced "usual, customary" fees.[11]

PHYSICIAN PAYMENT REFORM

In an effort to contain costs, government officials are seeking to change the way physicians caring for Medicare patients are paid.[12] During a congressional hearing addressing physician payment reform on May 24, 1988, Congressman Pete Stark (D-Calif.), chairman of the Subcommittee on Health of the Ways and Means Committee, said that any proposal for physician payment reform must reduce Medicare's spiraling outlays or "Congress will be forced by budgetary pressures to respond with a new round of freezes and cuts."[13]

Medicare and Medicaid accounted for 25 percent of individual physicians' practice income, according to a 1981 study. Survey results indicated that Medicare alone paid an average of $27,490 per physician.[14]

In addressing the subcommittee, William Roper, head of the Health Care Financing Administration (HCFA), listed several fundamental goals by which any proposal to reform Medicare physician payment policy should be evaluated:

1. to improve efficiency and establish fairer relative prices;

2. to provide incentives for appropriate utilization and cost containment;

3. to help assure that high quality and effective medical care is delivered while discouraging ineffective treatments; and

4. to assure that beneficiaries have access to services.[13]

Although Roper endorsed capitation as the best mode of ensuring Medicare (Part B) physician payment reform, the HCFA, with the AMA acting as subcontractor, had already contracted with Harvard University in September 1985 to construct a resource-cost-based relative-value scale for physician services. Mandated by Congress, the resource-based relative-value scale (RBRVS) study was conducted by the Harvard School of Public Health under the direction of economist William C. Hsiao and internist Peter Braun. The scale is described as resource-based because it measure the resource costs such as time, effort, training, and relative practice costs that are implicit in a physician's treatment of a patient. The new RBRVS will cross specialty boundaries to establish a single set of rankings for over 4,000 procedures and services in eighteen different specialties.[15]

Given the pressure to reduce health care expenditures and the high level of interest in changing the relative amounts paid for the performance of procedures, some version of the resource-based relative-value scale may supplant the UCR system as a means of determining physician reimbursement.

A resource-based fee schedule would decrease the average income of some specialists and increase that of others. The RBRVS is likely to boost fees for cognitive services (e.g., history taking, consultations, and physical exams), while reducing reimbursement for the high-tech specialties. Primary care physicians stand to gain from the study's results. The proceduralists whose income would suffer most would probably include surgeons, radiologists, and urologists.[15]

When asked to predict which specialties will suffer most economically should the scale be implemented, Braun replied that physicians should realize that they provide a mixture of services. Using surgeons' activities as an example, he pointed out that while surgeons are undercompensated for management, evaluation, consultation, and nonsurgical examination of patients, they may be relatively overpaid for their procedural activities.[16]

Although cost containment may be the primary objective of government officials who support the study, the RBRVS alone may not reduce Part B's total payments for physicians' services. In his statement before the subcommittee, Roper suggested the following:

While an RVS might help to correct some of the perceived inequities on the price side, the critical issue of volume and intensity will remain, as with any fee schedule. Moreover, income redistributions resulting from an RVS could exacerbate the Part B volume and intensity problem if physicians respond to fee reductions by increasing their volume and intensity of services.[13]

Volume and intensity increases, according to Roper, are the consequences of the new services and technology that have been developed over the last decade. Citing studies of geographic variation in the utilization of services, he noted that although newly developed services have provided substantial benefits for patients, physicians are guilty of "considerable unnecessary utilization of services."

If Roper's assessment is accurate, the implementation of the RBRVS will trigger overutilization of procedures, while failing to reduce spiraling Medicare Part B costs. Alternatively, when predicting the impact of changing the current Medicare policy of physician reimbursement, Glen Hammons, Robert Brook, and Joseph Newhouse emphasize that physicians are ethically bound to consider only the patient's interests when making patient care decisions and to disregard their own financial or other interests.[12] In an article urging physicians to alter their practices in preparation for "inevitable" reimbursement policy changes, Eugene Ogrod and Robert Doherty conclude that only physicians who are less than four years from retirement can afford to ignore changes in physician payment.[16]

Although practicing physicians will be primarily affected by alterations in the existing payment system, changes in reimbursement will undoubtedly affect medical students' specialty and subspecialty choices. Economic incentives that attract medical students to careers in certain specialties have been well documented. Thomas Dial and Paul Elliott cite two observations that had been noted in earlier investigations:

1. High degrees of indebtedness motivate students to select more lucrative specialties.

2. High degrees of indebtedness lead students to choose specialties requiring minimum training periods.[17]

Both the Dial and Elliott study and a study conducted by Gloria Bazzoli[18] suggest that debt has its most significant impact on medical student career choice when it is unsubsidized. For example, a Health Education Assistance Loan (HEAL) accrues interest through medical school and the postgraduate training period, but does not require the initial payment until the physician enters practice.

Having examined response trends evident in the Association of American Medical Colleges' Graduate Questionnaires of 1981 through 1986,[19] Cynthia Tudor noted a declining interest in primary care specialties, which particularly affected general internal medicine. Of 1981 graduates 43 percent selected primary care specialties (i.e., family practice, general internal medicine, general obstetrics-gynecology, and general pediatrics), but of the 1986 graduates only 36.6 percent expressed similar intentions. Of the primary care specialties, general internal medicine accounted for the greatest decrease in interest, dropping from 12.7 percent (1981) to 8.3 percent (1986).

In addition, a decreasing percentage of students surveyed between 1981 and 1986 were able to graduate without incurring debt. In 1986, 17 percent of medical graduates reported debt exceeding $50,000, compared with 2 percent in 1981. Using 1986 dollars, the average debt rose from $19,687 in 1981 to $33,499 in 1986.[19]

Having studied the responses of ninety-two members of the graduating class of 1983 at the University of Rochester School of Medicine, Robert Geertsma and John Romano concluded that there is a positive correlation between indebtedness and subspecialization.[20] The investigators also report that the more heavily indebted student is more likely to choose full-time private practice.

Data released in the 1987 National Study of Internal Medicine Manpower reveal that the subspecialization rate in internal medicine has declined from a high of 75 percent in 1977 to 53 percent in 1985. The largest internal medicine fellowship training programs in 1985–1986 were in cardiology, gastroenterology, and pulmonary disease—all representing procedure-oriented internal medicine subspecialties.[21]

Richard Lewis of the University of Colorado School of Medicine suggests that the apparent swing in doctors' interests reflects "not a shift from primary care toward the technological subspecialties, but one from the internal medicine subspecialties to the relatively less overcrowded technological subspecialties" (p. 453).[22] Lewis attributed young doctors' perceptions of surpluses to the "overcrowding laments" of their medical school role models as well as to the projections of the GMENAC report.

Like general internists, general surgeons are concerned that their specialty will suffer from declining interest. According to a study conducted in July 1985, only 25 percent of 625 chief surgical residents surveyed plan a practice limited to general surgery. When publishing their results, Ralph Greco and his colleagues voiced concern that the future of general surgery will be endangered since "[o]nly 12 percent of our future academic surgeons plan to practice general surgery."[23]

According to the survey's results, those doctors trained in independent programs (i.e., those programs that are not the primary surgical residency of an accredited U.S. medical school) are more likely to practice general surgery and are more likely to practice in smaller rural and suburban hospitals than are their university-trained counterparts. Consequently, independently trained general surgeons are less likely to assume teaching responsibilities. The authors are concerned that "[u]niversity training programs produce the future academic surgeons who are usually subspecialists and will in the future serve as role models for generations of subspecialists." Like Lewis, Greco and his colleagues assert that the decision to subspecialize is prompted by residents' perceptions of oversupply and is pursued because the doctors hope to gain an advantage in a highly competitive marketplace.[23]

EMERGING PRESSURES ON REIMBURSEMENT

If alterations are made in Medicare and other third-party payment systems through the implementation of some RBRVS schedule, physician reimbursement may ostensibly be more equitable, but reduced overall to diminish Medicare outlays. One must wonder if the quality of care will suffer as a result of such an alteration. Will medicine suffer because many potential American students will seek more lucrative professions, or will the medical profession be improved as the more altruistic and dedicated students pursue careers in medicine? If the government is successful in reducing physicians' income, will officials be receptive to medical students confronted with mounting educational costs and the prospect of reduced incomes?

Although controversy regarding payment mechanisms has persisted for over one hundred years, discussion continues. New factors that will influence future reimbursement include skyrocketing tuition and malpractice costs, an oversupply of physicians in some specialties and in some geographical areas, growing legislative pressure to further limit health expenditures, and an explosion of new procedures and techniques (including heart, liver, and bone marrow transplantation, lithotripters, and MRI scans).

In contrast to the physician-run health insurance plans of the 1920s, future directions of physician reimbursement will probably be established by Congress and state legislatures, with private health insurance companies following their lead. Responding to increasing budget pressure, Congress will incorporate new mechanisms for determining physician reimbursement. A form of the resource-based relative-value scale is now part of these inevitable changes in Medicare Part B and physician fees generated through Medicaid. The impact of these changes on career choices made by undergraduate and medical students remains to be seen. What has already been demonstrated in recent years is that the number of medical school students, internal medicine residents, and subspecialty fellows has declined.

Little imagination is required to appreciate why a bright college graduate would balk at the prospect of accumulating a $100,000 debt followed by six years with a subsistence salary to face uncertain income, no matter how exciting the subspecialty. It will be Congress' challenge to pay for a reasonable standard of health care, while maintaining a fee schedule sufficient to attract young physicians into specialties and subspecialties.

NOTES

1. Carl J. Schramm, *Health Care and Its Costs* (New York: W. W. Norton, 1987).

2. Paul Starr. *The Social Transformation of America and Medicine* (New York: Basic Books, 1982).

3. Marshall W. Raffel, *The U.S. Health System* (New York: John Wiley & Sons, 1984).

4. D. McCarthy, "Why Are Today's Medical Students Choosing High-Technology Specialties over Internal Medicine?" *New England Journal of Medicine* 317 (1987): 567–69.

5. A. Owens, "Doctors' Earnings: On the Rise Again," *Medical Economics* (September 7, 1987): 212–37.

6. M. Kirchner, "Are Doctors Pushing Fees to the Breaking Point?" *Medical Economics* (October 5, 1987): 152–67.

7. American Society of Internal Medicine, *Seven Years Later: ASIM's Chronology of the Cognitive Services Concept* (American Society of Internal Medicine, 1988).

8. W. Sobaski, director of the Division of Reimbursement and Economic Studies, Office of Research and Development, Health Care Financing Administration, telephone interview, August 1988.

9. T. C. Delbanco, K. C. Meyers, and E. A. Sengal, "Paying the Physician's Fee: Blue Shield and the Reasonable Charge." *New England Journal of Medicine* 301 (1979): 1314–20.

10. L. Gregory Pawlson, acting chairman of the Department of Health Care Sciences at The George Washington University, personal interview, August 1988.

11. Omnibus Budget Reconciliation Act (OBRA) of 1987, Part 2, p. 823.

12. G. T. Hammons, R. H. Brook, and J. P. Newhouse, "Changing Physician Payment for Medicare Patients: Projected Effects on the Quality of Care," *Western Journal of Medicine* (1986): 704–9.

13. Subcommittee on Health, House Ways and Means Committee, May 31, 1988.

14. A. Owens, "How Much of Your Money Comes from Third Parties?" *Medical Economics* (April 4, 1983): 254–63.

15. M. Kirchner, "Will This Formula Change the Way You Get Paid?" *Medical Economics* (April 4, 1988): 138–52.

16. E. S. Ogrod and R. B. Doherty, "Enhanced Reimbursement Is Becoming a Reality," *Consultant* 28 (1988): 89–95.

17. T. H. Dial and P. R. Elliott, "Relationship of Scholarships and Indebtedness to Medical Students' Career Plans," *Journal of Medical Education* 62 (1987): 316–24.

18. G. J. Bazzoli, "Medical Education Indebtedness: Does It Affect Physicians' Specialty Choice?" *Health Affairs* (Summer 1985): 98–104.

19. C. Tudor, "Career Plans and Debt Levels of Graduating U.S. Medical Students, 1981–1986," *Journal of Medical Education* 63 (1988): 271–75.

20. R. H. Geertsma and J. Romano, "Relationship Between Expected Indebtedness and Career Choice of Medical Students," *Journal of Medical Education* 61 (1986): 555–59.

21. M. W. Cox et al., "National Study of Internal Medicine Manpower: XI. Internal Medicine Residency and Fellowship Training in the 1980's," *Annals of Internal Medicine* 106 (1987): 734–40.

22. R. Lewis, "Letter to the Editor," *New England Journal of Medicine* 318 (1988): 453.

23. R. S. Greco, A. P. Donetz, R. E. Brolin, S. Z. Trooskin, and J. W. MacKenzie, "The Influence of Debt, Moonlighting, Practice, Oversupply and Gender on Career Development of Residents in University and Independent Training Programs," *Surgery, Gynecology and Obstetrics* 165 (1987): 19–24.

11

Nurse Practitioners and Physician Assistants: Revenue and Reimbursement

Jean Johnson and James F. Cawley

Viewed overall, the creation of nurse practitioners (NPs) and physician assistants (PAs) represents a significant shift in the division of medical labor in this country. Prior to their inception, the clinical domain of diagnosis and treatment belonged solely to the physician. With the advent of these clinicians (sometimes collectively termed midlevel health practitioners or nonphysician health providers), new patterns of medical practice emerged, incorporating these providers in many types of practices and settings. The practice of these providers has raised questions about how they would be paid. Even after NPs and PAs have been in existence for twenty-five years, issues regarding reimbursement for their services are not fully resolved.

The parallel development of the roles of the NPs and PAs was rooted in the social context of the 1960s and stemmed from the then widely held perception that the United States needed additional primary care health manpower. For PAs the role initially provided military corpsmen returning from Vietnam an entre into clinical positions in the civilian health sector. Nurses found that the NP role allowed expansion of their clinical skills with greater autonomy and responsibility. The clear potential of NPs and PAs to increase access to primary health care was coupled with the social mandate of remedying the severe maldistribution of health care services existent at that time.

The notion that NPs and PAs could become effective providers of primary care, begun as an experiment in health manpower, has proved to be enormously successful. Extensive research over the past twenty-five years has shown that NPs and PAs are well accepted by patients and by physicians, provide a high quality of care, and are clinically effective in a wide variety of practice settings.[1] An additional factor in their success has been the economic rationality of their utilization. NPs and PAs have training costs and salaries far below those of physicians; yet careful studies show that they can manage up to 80 percent of the medical duties required in a primary care practice.[2] These characteristics have fueled the steady growth and continuing demand for NPs and PAs. There are presently over 20,000 nurse practitioners and approximately 22,000 physician assistants in full-time clinical practice.

The utilization of NPs and PAs has increased during a time when some have suggested that there is little need for such health providers. This position is taken mainly because of projections of a physician surplus. According to the now questionable GMENAC report, estimates of overall physician manpower indicate the supply could exceed the need by 1992.[3] It would appear from current trends that this may not occur, and that the rapid increase in the number of physicians in the early 1980s has had no dampening effect on the employment of NPs and PAs. In fact, the demand for NPs and PAs in the medical marketplace has never been stronger. As their traditional roles as primary care providers in family practices, outpatient clinics, rural practices, HMOs, and ambulatory health facilities have become better established, new roles have also developed from these in specialty and subspecialty practices, frequently in inpatient settings. Numerous positions, particularly for PAs, have emerged as hospital house staff on medical, surgical, and pediatric services. In these settings, PAs and NPs function on the level of a first-year resident, performing a wide variety of medical tasks and procedures and working with senior residents and attending physicians.[4]

An important element in their viability currently lies in the economics of practice. While there is not a totally homogeneous picture of NP and PA practice, some generalizations can be made. Economic viability depends primarily on practice-setting characteristics. Determining factors include the type of organization or practice structure, prevailing physician reimbursement levels, the willingness of physicians to delegate tasks, the productivity of the NP or PA as measured by income generated from patient visits, and the overhead costs of having an NP and a PA to provide services.

PRACTICE SETTINGS AND EMPLOYMENT

While early practice patterns and much of the published literature examining NPs and PAs focus on the primary care setting, NPs and PAs today work at all levels of health care in a wide variety of settings. A national survey of pediatric NPs, for example, revealed that 22 percent of the respondents worked in hospitals, 20 percent in community health agencies, 17 percent in private pediatricians' offices, 10 percent in specialty clinics, 6 percent in health maintenance organizations (HMOs), and the rest mainly in nursing schools and military clinics.[5] NPs are also increasingly being employed in home health agencies and in geriatric facilities.[6, 7] Both NPs and PAs are being increasingly utilized in primary care walk-in clinics, industrial clinics, correctional institutions, and university health centers.[8]

Different types of practice settings have different implications for any economic analysis of the benefits of hiring NPs or PAs. For example, comparing NPs with other nurses might be more appropriate than comparing NPs with physicians in such settings as home health agencies, HMOs, schools, and businesses—that is, places where NPs might be employed instead of, or in addition to, registered or licensed practical nurses. In these settings, the NPs—the more costly alternative—might be selected because they could provide a wider range of services. However, an NP is not always more costly than another nurse. In a 1984 study, a clinical nurse specialist with an M.S.N. degree commanded about $2,000 more than an NP with an M.S.N.[9] NPs employed in schools, for example, can serve as liaisons among the various health care providers serving the schools; NPs can also provide backup support and in-house education to school nurses and provide educational services to teachers, parents, and students.[10]

Because of increases in the variety of settings in which NPs work, their employment rates might reasonably be expected to be higher than ever. However, proportionately fewer NPs are working as nurse practitioners in the 1980s than were doing so in the 1970s.[11] The extent to which this decrease reflects either increased competition from the growing supply of physicians or the fact that NPs are moving into positions that are not considered NP positions, but in which NP skills are significantly utilized, is not known.

PAs also work in a wide variety of settings and in every level of health care from primary to tertiary. Of all PAs, about one-third work in office-based practices (about half of these PAs work with physicians in solo practices), another one-third or so based in hospitals, and the remaining one-third work in prepaid groups, public health departments, drug and alcohol rehabilitation centers, industrial settings, nursing homes, prisons and jails, and military facilities.[12] Considerable change has occurred in the proportion of PAs employed in various settings. For example, the proportion of PAs employed in hospitals grew from 10 percent in 1974 to well over 30 percent in 1990 (American Academy of Physician Assistants, data on file).

Increasing numbers of NPs, as well as PAs, are finding work in hospitals. This development may or may not be related to the implementation of prospective payment for hospitals based on diagnosis-related groups (DRGs). In fact, it may be occurring despite DRGs. Not only did this trend predate DRGs, but also it is more likely to be related to the growth in the supply of physicians, increasing medical specialization, and the cost-effectiveness of NP and PA practices.

As the number of physicians increases in certain specialties (e.g., surgery), residency positions are being decreased to contain the numbers, and PAs are being employed as "junior house staff" to supplement patient care.[4]

New employment opportunities for NPs and PAs may also stem from the trend among hospitals to establish community-based ambulatory care centers in order to broaden their patient bases and to assure themselves of solid sources of inpatient referrals. Hospital managers recognize that their best interests are served by providing these services as efficiently as possible by employing NPs and PAs.

PAYMENT FOR SERVICES

In the 1970s a major reason cited by physicians as a disincentive to employing an NP or a PA was the lack of reimbursement at either the federal or the state level or through private third-party payers.[13] Many observers felt that providing coverage for NP and PA services within medical practices would increase incentives for physicians in fee-for-service practices to employ these providers. Prevailing coverage and payment for NP and PA services would increase practice revenues for employing physicians, particularly if the physician billed the carrier at the prevailing (M.D.) rate. Recognition by Medicare or other insurers of the legitimate clinical services provided in a practice by an NP or a PA at a rate somewhat less than that of the physician would offer a means whereby the incentive to employ an NP or a PA would be maintained and, at the same time, be acceptable to third-party payers since their costs for the provision of a given service could be less.

The vast majority of NPs and PAs work as salaried employees of either a private practice (solo or group) health care institution or agency. In private practice, billing is done primarily under physician authorization and is paid directly to the practice. Increasingly, carriers have begun to provide coverage for NP and PA services in certain settings where it is explicitly designated that the NP or PA provided the service. In the hospital setting, services provided by PAs are covered at 75 percent of the physician rate under Medicare Part B, a provision in place since 1987. No similar rubric covers NP services. In the HMO setting, most NP and PA services are covered through the capitated financing of care. HMOs have an incentive for hiring NPs and PAs since their practice is recognized and is less costly to the HMO system.

The average salary for an NP or a PA in 1989 was estimated to be $30,000 to $32,000 per year plus employee benefits. Salary and benefits depend somewhat on the type of practice, the number of hours worked, and the geographical region. NPs or PAs working in a neurology practice usually have a higher salary than those working for Planned Parenthood or a community health agency. Many NPs and PAs who work on a call basis—for example, those in surgical practices—may earn considerably more with the overtime differential. Many NPs and PAs who work in a private individual or group practice may receive retirement benefits, pension and/or profit-sharing benefits, and other benefits such as paid professional organization dues and allowances for continuing education conferences.

INCOME GENERATION VERSUS COST

Since payment for NP and PA services is strongly linked to physician reimbursement, and since NP and PA practice characteristics most resemble those of family practitioners and internists, the relationships of NP and PA service provision in these types of practices will be considered. The type of physician practice will directly affect reimbursement levels for NP or PA services. According to American Medical Association (AMA) data, family physicians receive less per patient visit for both new and established patients, so that an NP or a PA working for an internist will generate a higher revenue than one working for a general practitioner.[14] The AMA data indicate that internists, at least since 1976, have received a 45 percent higher reimbursement rate than have family practitioners. In 1986 internists received a mean reimbursement rate of $34.03, while family practitioners received a mean rate of $23.48 for an established patient. In that same year the mean fee for an office visit to an internist for a new patient was $79.19, as compared to less than half that amount, $34.61, for a visit to a family practitioner. Obviously, an NP or a PA working for an internist will be able to generate a higher income for the practice than will one working with a general practitioner.

Table 11.1 displays potential profitability rations of NPs and PAs over time, given the differences in payment rates for family practitioners and internists. Average salaries are used for each type of provider. Benefits were calculated equally at a rate of 20 percent of salary. This model assumes that an NP or a PA will be engaged in activities beyond direct patient contact, such as returning patient calls and calling for test results. Only salary and benefits are included as cost factors in this comparison, assuming that both types of practices would incur similar overhead costs (such as additional office space). The profitability ratios have increased in both settings since 1976.

Income generated is based on a model in which an NP or a PA sees seventy-two patients per week for forty-seven weeks per year. In addition to NPs and PAs being profitable, the profitability ratio using NPs and PAs has increased for both physician groups over time. This suggests that while the ability to generate income has increased due to increasing reimbursement rates, NP and PA salaries and benefits have not increased at the same rate as their income-generating ability. Income generated after salary and benefits has increased two and a half times since 1976, whereas salary and benefits have increased approximately one and a half times.

Some argue that NPs and PAs are not as attractive as they once were, particularly with the fear on the part of physicians that jobs may become

Table 11.1
Profitability Ratio

	Cost to the Practice of NP/PA Salary & Benefits	Income Generated by NP/PA—Family Practice[a]	Income to Internist, Generated by NP/NA—Practice[b]	Profitability Ratio for Family Practice	Profitability Ratio for Internist Practice
1976	21,960	36,683	55,768	1.67	2.54
1978	24,400[c]	42,571	59,491	1.74	2.44
1982	29,280	63,619	96,619	2.17	3.30
1984	31,720[d]	70,523	109,322	2.22	3.45
1986	35,380	81,351	122,805	2.30	3.47

Source: American Medical Association, *Socioeconomic Characteristics of Medical Practice* (1987).

[a]American Medical Association, Center for Health Policy Research, *Socioeconomic Characteristics of Medical Practice* (Chicago: American Medical Association, 1987).

[b]Based on mean physician fees for an office visit with an established patient (American Medical Association, *Characteristics of Medical Practice*).

[c]H. A. Sultz et al., "Nurse Practitioners: A Decade of Change—Part IV," *Nursing Outlook* 32 (1984): 158–63.

[d]U.S. Department of Health and Human Services, *The Registered Nurse Population, Findings from the National Sample Survey of Registered Nurses* (Springfield, Va.: 1986).

scarce and that income levels will decrease because of increased competition. There are reports of physicians competing directly with NPs and PAs for salaried positions in HMOs in certain large urban areas. There is, however, little indication that there is unemployment in the physician community. Furthermore, the Physician Payment Review Commission notes that there is no sign of decreasing physician salaries overall.[15] In fact, between 1975 and 1987 the mean net income of all physicians more than doubled. In real dollar terms, after adjusting for inflation, physicians' net income rose by 13 percent, while that of the average full-time U.S. employee increased by only 3 percent. In analyzing 1986 NP, PA, and physician salaries, there continued to be significant differences in salary levels. As shown in Table 11.2, these differences are most marked for NP and PA salaries when compared to that of internists. Whereas the 1984 mean income of family practitioners after expenses and before taxes was nearly three times the mean income of an NP or a PA, the mean income of internists was nearly four times that of NPs and PAs. Of course, much of this salary differential should be expected, based on the difference in the cost and length of education for each of these providers. The rate of return to investment in education is directly reflected in potential earnings. Based on estimates of education costs made by the Congressional Budget Office in 1979 and assuming a 6 percent annual increase in the cost of education, the education of an NP in 1986 would be $15,476; that of a PA, $17,914; and that of an M.D., $91,266.[13] The cost of education of an M.D. is approximately five to six times that of an NP or a PA. There is clearly a relationship between rate of return on investment and earnings.

Assuming that rates of clinical productivity of NPs and PAs are about three-fourths those of physicians, the educational costs and resultant lower earnings of NPs and PAs suggest that these providers could have a significant impact on holding down health care costs. Indeed, this position was one of the critical reasons for the creation of the professions. But there have been several significant barriers to this becoming a reality.

Even though NPs and PAs can theoretically charge patients less for their services, traditionally this has been the exception rather than the rule. Most NPs and PAs work in settings in which the charge for their services is at physician rates. This makes utilization of an NP or a PA cost effective to a physician practice, but the benefit is usually not passed on to society. This has been true in office-based practices, as well as in institutional practices in which there is physician billing. True cost-effectiveness to society from utilization of these providers can occur in practice settings such as prepaid health plans (HMOs) in which premiums can be held down because costs are based, in part, on salary levels of the providers, rather than on M.D. reimbursement rates. The role that NPs and PAs can play in prepaid health plans, including both HMOs and independent practitioner associations (IPAs) is increasingly important. Enrollment in HMOs has increased from

Table 11.2
Income Ratio Approximation

	NP/PA[a]	General Practitioner[b]	Internist[b]	Income Ratio for Family Practice	Income Ratio for Internist Practice
1978	20,000[c]	53,700	62,500	2.69	3.13
1982	24,000	71,400	86,900	2.98	3.62
1984	26,000[d]	71,600	104,200	2.75	4.01
1986	29,000	80,300	109,400	2.77	3.77

Source: American Medical Association, *Socioeconomic Characteristics of Medical Practice* (1987).

[a]American Medical Association, Center for Health Policy Research, *Socioeconomic Characteristics of Medical Practice* (Chicago: American Medical Association, 1987).

[b]All incomes calculated without benefits included.

[c]Adjusted from salary data from H. A. Sultz et al., "Nurse Practitioners: A Decade of Change—Part IV," *Nursing Outlook* 32 (1984): 158–63.

[d]U.S. Department of Health and Human Services, *The Registered Nurse Population, Findings from the National Sample Survey of Registered Nurses* (Springfield, Va.: 1986).

6 million in 1976 to over 28 million in 1987.[16] Hospital settings, in which many PAs are moving into house officer positions, may also be cost effective to society from several perspectives. As a house officer, a PA or an NP can provide continuity of care that enhances the quality of care delivered. In addition, there are signs that continued funding for physician residents through the Medicare "pass through" for medical education may be significantly decreased. PAs or NPs, rather than physicians, can be built into a cost center of the hospital as permanent employees and thus have their services billed and reimbursed at a rate lower than attending physician rates.

REGULATION OF PRACTICE

The practice of billing for NP and PA services at the physician rate is based in the continued control by physicians of these practitioners. By law, physician assistant practice is controlled by the physician. PAs practice under state medical practice acts which mandate that physician assistants be supervised by a physician.

NPs practice under state nurse practice acts, with the board of nursing in each state defining the scope of NP practices. Even with the definition of practice being largely determined by nursing, few NPs practice independently. NPs have not practiced independently for two major reasons. First, most NPs recognize the need for collaborating with physicians for consultation and referral. An important aspect of the NP role is knowing when a problem is beyond the NP's scope of practice. In addition, the third-party payer system, with one exception, will reimburse for services only if there is physician supervision. This means that physicians must countersign orders and progress notes within some established time frame. An increasingly common model of practice regulations within states requires that an NP have a written agreement with a physician who will provide consultation and referral services. Many states also have the requirement for a written protocol that is established jointly by a physician and an NP.

POLICY INITIATIVES

There have been several initiatives to facilitate the promise of NPs and PAs in providing access to high-quality, lower-cost care. The first came in 1977 with the passage of the Rural Health Clinics Act. This legislation provided both Medicare and Medicaid reimbursement to NPs and PAs who delivered care in federally certified rural health clinics. The reimbursement was paid to the clinic and was based on the cost of services provided. This method of payment created a financial disincentive because of the frequently long wait for payment. Charges could be submitted only after care was delivered, and many providers could not carry the costs of operating clinics for a prolonged period of time.

In addition to reimbursement for NP and PA services, the Rural Health Clinics Act also allows for ownership of a clinic by a PA or an NP. The provision relating to this states that "the physician assistant or nurse practitioner member of the staff may be the owner of the clinic or an employee of the clinic." This provision has been rarely used. There are increasing congressional efforts to support the practice of NPs and PAs in the rural areas. This effort is due to the recognition that rural health needs are still not being met fully. For example, in 1987 the Health Care Financing Administration (HFCA) projected that by 1990 there would be 2,000 certified rural health clinics.[17] However, in 1988 there were only 426 such clinics. As of January 1989 physician assistant services provided in rural health manpower shortage areas may be reimbursed through Medicare Part B without the need for certification of the clinic as a rural health clinic. There is no similar provision for nurse practitioners.

Another governmental action intended to expand NP services was the legislative recognition of direct reimbursement for NPs through the Civilian Health and Medical Program of the Uniformed Services (CHAMPUS). An NP in any practice setting could bill for services provided to a CHAMPUS member, provided that the NP obtained a billing number from the fiscal intermediary that serviced the area in which the practice was located. During the period from May 1980 to March 1981 in which CHAMPUS kept data on NP charges, few claims were actually generated by NPs. By March 1981, only 54 total claims had been submitted for reimbursement by seven nurses in four states.[18] CHAMPUS no longer separates claims by provider type, so there is no current information on billing. It was felt that the number of claims was low because few NPs were aware of how to obtain a provider number and because most NPs are salaried and thus do not feel a need to bill for their services. To date, CHAMPUS has been primarily paying for NP services; however, PA services are eligible as well.

An area of practice in which NPs and PAs could make a significant contribution to patient care, as well as to cost savings, is in caring for the elderly. The over-65 age group currently comprises about 12 percent of the population and will increase to 22 percent of the population by 2050, with the graying of the baby boom generation.[19] The most dramatic increase will be in the 75-and-older age group. The 75-and-older age group utilizes health services to a greater extent than any other age group does. Medicare expenditures have increased an average of 13.1 percent per year from 1980 to 1988 and in 1988 federal outlays for Medicare were approximately $88 billion. Medicare Part B expenditures are increasing the most rapidly, and physician services account for about 72 percent of Part B outlays.[20] Analysis of the Medicare data suggests that the increase in spending for physician services is due mainly to an increase in the volume of services per beneficiary and the substitution of more expensive services for less expensive services.

Many options will have to be examined to develop reasonable strategies for containing costs. Among these strategies could be enabling NPs and PAs to provide care to this elderly population at a rate that is reimbursed at less than the physician rate. In 1986 approximately $7.4 billion of Medicare Part B funds was spent on services provided in a physician's office; $833 million was spent on intermediate service and $785 million on limited office medical services.[20]

These amounts do not include hospital medical services or outpatient surgical procedures. The types of services provided during these visits are most likely to be related to the management of chronic diseases, which NPs and PAs are well trained to do. If NPs and PAs provided only 20 percent of intermediate and limited services at a reimbursement rate of 75 percent of physician charges, over $80 million could be saved in health care costs. A recent initiative to reimburse PA services through Medicare Part B was enacted under the Omnibus Budget Reconciliation Act of 1986 which authorizes payment to the PA for providing "physician services" in a hospital, skilled nursing facility, or intermediate care facility or for assisting in surgery. The PA must be supervised by the physician, but supervision is defined by state law and does not necessarily require direct on-site supervision as Medicare has required in the past to reimburse for both NP and PA services. Reimbursement is indirect (made to the practice, not the PA) and is graded on a scale depending on the practice setting. For example, PAs assisting in surgery are reimbursed at 65 percent of the physician rate, in hospitals at 75 percent, and in nursing homes at 85 percent.

The area of practice in which NPs and PAs have the most potential for having a profound positive impact is in nursing homes. There has been much interest in enabling NPs and PAs to practice in nursing homes. However, this area of practice has been limited by requirements established by the HCFA that demand direct supervision of practice and at times have not recognized the legitimacy of NP and PA practice within the nursing home setting at all.

Recent data show that of the 23,600 nursing homes, approximately 250 have NPs on staff.[21] The proportion of PAs working in nursing homes has been about 5 percent and has remained stable since 1981.[22] The HCFA has been critical of physician participation in the care of nursing home residents, believing that M.D.s do not provide the kind of medical leadership in this area that is necessary. Thus, the HCFA has been fearful that enabling the practice of NPs and PAs would further separate physicians from nursing homes. However, with broad-based support from physician groups, consumers, and the nursing home industry, the HCFA has included in its Notice of Final Rules (*Federal Register*, February 1989) provisions to recognize NP and PA services provided in nursing homes. These regulations will require M.D.s to do admission histories, physical examinations, and orders. The NP or PA can make visits for acute problems and can make every other routine visit, alternating with physicians. In addition, there is no requirement for direct on-site physician supervision. At this time, the billing mechanism or reimbursement rate has not been established.

TOWARD THE FUTURE

Nurse practitioners and physician assistants have become safely established in the structure of the health delivery system. They have proven their worth over twenty-five years of careful evaluation. The trend, as indicated, is toward increasing recognition of their contribution to medical care through multiple funding mechanisms for their services. This trend is partly due to the need to separate NP and PA payment from physician payment, so that for the benefits of cost savings from their practices accrue to society and not only to physician practices.

Nurse practitioners and physician assistants have succeeded because they have filled a clear niche in American health care. They provide a wide range of medical and health care tasks from the most elementary to the very complex. Estimates of the tasks that NPs and PAs can perform range from 70 to 80 percent of the physicians capabilities with no diminution in quality of care. In some instances, probably because of their increased emphasis on interpersonal skills and patient education, NPs and PAs perform some clinical services even better than M.D.s.

The use of NPs and PAs in medical practice has taught policymakers several lessons in terms of the rational utilization of health manpower. NPs and PAs can provide a significant number of medical care services at a cost considerably less than that of physicians. Their proved effectiveness in medical care has exploded the "myth of physician necessity"—that is, the belief that a physician needs to be present for every illness.[4] Patient acceptance of these providers has always been quite high. In a large number of instances, NPs and PAs function in roles originally hoped for in their creation—spending more time with patients, engaging in patient education and health counselling, and bringing a more humanistic approach to primary medical care. These attributes are being increasingly appreciated by employing physicians and patients alike. These practice capabilities, coupled with their solid background in medical science and technological skills, will keep these practitioners in high demand throughout the next decade.

NOTES

1. U.S. Congress, Office of Technology Assessment, *Nurse Practitioners, Physician Assistants and Certified Nurse-Midwives: A Policy Analysis*, Health Technology Case Study 37, OTA-HCS–37 (Washington, D.C.: U.S. Government Printing Office, 1986).

2. J. C. Record et al., "New Health Professionals After a Decade and a Half: Delegation, Productivity and Costs in Primary Care," *Journal of Health Politics, Policy and Law* 5 (1980): 470–97.

3. U.S. Department of Health and Human Services, Public Health Service, Health Resources and Services Administration, *Fifth Report to the President and Congress on the Status of Health Personnel in the United States* (Washington, D.C.: U.S. Government Printing Office, 1986).

4. G. E. Schafft and J. F. Cawley, *Physician Assistants in a Changing Health Care Environment* (Rockville, Md.: Aspen, 1988).

5. K. Mitchell, "NAPNAPs Scope of Practice Survey: Results, Revisions, and Issues," *Pediatric Nursing* 9 (1983): 199–203.

6. S. R. Gambert et al., "Role of the Physician-Extender in the Long Term Care Setting," *Wisconsin Medical Journal* 82:9 (1983): 30–32.

7. J. L. Weston, *NPs and PAs: Changes—Where, Whether and Why* (Washington, D.C.: National Center for Health Services Research, 1984).

8. M. M. Manber, "NPs, MDs and PAs: Meshing Their Changing Roles," *Medical World News* 26 (1985): 53–71.

9. U.S. Department of Health and Human Services, *The Registered Nurse Population, Findings from the National Sample Survey of Registered Nurses* (Springfield, Va.: 1986).

10. S. D. Sobolewski, "Cost-Effective School Nurse Practitioner Services," *Journal of School Health* 51 (1981): 585–88.

11. H. A. Sultz et al., "Nurse Practitioners: A Decade of Change—Part IV," *Nursing Outlook* 32 (1984): 158–63.

12. American Academy of Physician Assistants, *1987 Master File Survey of Physician Assistants* (Arlington, Va.: AAPA, 1987).

13. U.S. Congress, Congressional Budget Office, *Physician Extenders: Their Current and Future Roles in Medical Care Delivery* (Washington, D.C.: U.S. Government Printing Office, 1979).

14. American Medical Association, Center for Health Policy Research, *Socioeconomic Characteristics of Medical Practice* (Chicago: American Medical Association, 1987).

15. Physician Payment Review Commission, *Annual Report to Congress* (Washington, D.C.: U.S. Government Printing Office, 1989).

16. U.S. Bureau of the Census, *Statistical Abstract of the United States: 1989*, 109th ed. (Washington, D.C.: Government Printing Office, 1989).

17. D. Hardy, "Rural Health Clinics: Up for Ownership," *Journal of Pediatric Health Care* 2:3 (1988): 154–55.

18. J. Johnson, "The Champus Hoopla," *Nurse Practitioner* 7:6 (1982): 8–10.

19. U.S. Bureau of the Census, "Demographic and Socioeconomic Aspects of Aging in the United States," *Current Population Reports*, Ser. P–23, no. 138 (Washington, D.C.: Government Printing Office, 1984).

20. C. Hebling and R. Keen, "Use and Cost of Physician Services Under Medicare, 1986," *Health Care Financing Review* 10:3 (1989): 109–22.

21. P. Ebersole, "Gerontological Nurse Practitioners, Past and Present," *Geriatric Nursing* 6:4 (1985): 219–22.

22. American Academy of Physician Assistants, *1984 Physician Assistant Masterfile Survey* (Arlington, Va.: AAPA, 1984).

Part IV
Case Study: Medicare

Since it is impossible to discuss physician reimbursement in the United States without reference to Medicare, the previous chapters have touched on various aspects of the program. This final part takes a more systematic approach to an understanding of the nature of the Medicare program, the proposals for reform that have appeared over the years, and the public policy issues that have shaped its past and are now affecting its future.

Thus, James Bonanno Bautz reviews the Medicare reimbursement structure and the two prevalent reform alternatives of relative-value scales and prospective payment, concluding with an interesting comparison to Medicaid reimbursement. Edward Berkowitz and Wendy Wolff put this structure in a historical context, describing the competing congressional objectives that resulted in the series of compromises that made Medicare politically possible in the first place. They also note the historic ebb and flow of interest in the option of prospective reimbursement through contracted providers such as health maintenance organizations (HMOs). Finally, L. Gregory Pawlson joins the financing and historic perspectives in an effort to identify those techniques to limit the costs to Medicare of physician payment that stand some chance of success in terms of both politics and accounting.

Although the Medicare experience might at first strike the reader as one of much sound and fury and little form, in fact these chapters do turn on certain strikingly recurrent themes. One is that Medicare has been a resounding success, for its aim of providing a guarantee of acute health care to the elderly has surely been achieved. Yet Medicare also carried within it the seeds of its own failure, in the sense that it was designed with few barriers to increased cost. The reassurance this provided its beneficiaries in the short run threatens to destroy it in the long run.

Another impressive theme that recurs in these chapters is that the federal government, though responding fitfully to this threat, has steadily tried to become a less passive payer. Even with broad and deep agreement about the principle of a more aggressive posture with respect to provider charges, the future of Medicare reform in Congress is likely to resemble the past in its incrementalism, yet another theme stressed in these chapters. Further, one is impressed that Medicaid's well-known difficulties in achieving a decent level of health care delivery that is equitable from one state and region to another, as well as financially sound, have a great deal to do with its policy role in the shadow of Medicare.

Doubts about the long-range prospects of Medicare cost containment, given the essential structure of our medical-industrial complex, have led some recent commentators to urge that the elderly should themselves review the appropriateness of much of the care they receive. It is held that much intensive, technologically sophisticated intervention near the end of life is drastically inappropriate and burdensome for the patients themselves. Explicit rationing based on age or severity of illness or some combination of the two, particularly if endorsed by those who are patients or anticipate the status, would surely moderate demands on Medicare, though there is disagreement about its overall effect on health care costs. The resultant savings could then be redistributed to those who have a reasonable prospect of a longer future, but who are at risk for all sorts of debilitating morbidity, including especially those currently ineligible for Medicaid benefits who are nevertheless poor.

Some will say that this sort of talk demonstrates the bankrupt nature of a political system unable to come to terms with tough financing choices. Yet it seems fair to say that if textbook solutions to the Medicare reimbursement problem continue to fall short of their ends in the rough-and-tumble of legislative processes and administrative applications, we will have to seek more drastic solutions. Taken together, these chapters provide a road map that alerts us to the obstacles that lie behind as well as ahead of us. Whether past or future, these obstacles turn out to look remarkably familiar.

12

Medicare and Medicaid: The Government as Third-Party Payer

James Bonanno Bautz

Since the adoption of the Medicare program in 1954 and the Medicaid program shortly thereafter, the federal government has assumed an increasingly important role in physician reimbursement. Total U.S. expenditures for physician services increased from $8.5 billion in 1965 to $82.5 billion in 1985. The proportion of these expenditures contributed by the federal government under Medicare increased from 11 percent in 1970 to 21 percent in 1985, with federal/state Medicaid payments accounting for another 4 percent.[1] By 1988 direct physician payments under Medicare Part B had grown to $24 billion.

Medicare's influence on physician reimbursement goes well beyond its growing importance as paymaster. Medicare policies regarding physician reimbursement have had a major impact on the approach taken by Medicaid and private third-party payers, and the latter are likely to follow Medicare's lead in its current efforts to restructure physician reimbursement. After analyzing the present situation with regard to physician payment under Medicare, this chapter will examine various reforms in payment structures that are currently under consideration. The chapter will conclude with a brief discussion of parallel developments in the Medicaid system.

MEDICARE REIMBURSEMENT: DEVELOPMENT OF THE EXISTING "CUSTOMARY, PREVAILING, AND REASONABLE" STRUCTURE

In adopting the amendments to the Social Security Act that established Medicare (Title XVIII, "Health Insurance for the Aged") in 1965, Congress declared its intention of assuring elderly persons access to "comprehensive health services of high quality" without regard to economic status. Medicare Part A, financed from Social Security payroll taxes, provides coverage for hospital charges (traditionally on the basis of cost reimbursement) after payment of an initial deductible by the beneficiary. A supplementary plan under Medicare Part B, financed from beneficiary premiums, deductibles and copayments supplemented by general federal tax revenues, covers physician services on the basis of "customary, prevailing, and reasonable" (CPR) charges. Under this system, which was beginning to come into use in Blue Shield Plans at the time of Medicare's adoption, the private insurers administering the program as fiscal intermediaries for the government, are directed to:

Assure that, where payment . . . is on a charge basis, such charges will be reasonable and not higher than the charge applicable for a comparable service and under comparable circumstances to the policyholders and subscribers of the carrier. . . . In determining the reasonable charge . . . there shall be taken into consideration the physician's customary charge for similar services . . . as well as the prevailing charges in the locality for similar services.[2]

Thus, two screens, generally updated annually, are applied to a physician's actual charges. The customary charge screen reflects the median amount charged by the physician for the particular service in the preceding year. The prevailing charge screen is set at a certain percentile of charges (initially the ninetieth percentile, more recently closer to the seventy-fifth) for the particular service by peer physicians in the same specialty and locality during the previous year. Actual reimbursement by Medicare is then set at 80 percent of whichever is lowest of actual, customary, or prevailing charges, with patient copayments covering the other 20 percent. More recently, drawing on the statutory language, "inherent reasonableness" has begun to be applied as an additional screen to limit charges and will be discussed at greater length below.

In the early years of the Medicare program, the focus was on expanding access to medical care and encouraging physician participation in the program; reimbursement rates were generally close to actual charges. However, faced with dramatic cost escalations, Medicare soon began to tighten its reimbursement rules. The Social Security Act Amendments of 1972, which expanded Medicare to cover disabled patients and those with end-stage renal disease, also limited increases in the prevailing charge screen to the increase in the Medicare Economic Index, which is pegged to changes in workers' earning and physician office practice expenses. Efforts to control spiraling Medicare Part A costs led to Congress' adoption in 1983 of a new, prospectively determined reimbursement mechanism for hospitals based on discharge diagnosis, with 470 diagnosis-related groups (DRGs) listed. The Department of Health and Human Services (DHHS) was directed by Congress to study the feasibility of applying the DRG approach to physician reimbursement under Medicare Part B at a future date.[3]

With the substantial decline in Part A growth following the adoption of the DRG reimbursement system (from an annual average of 17.3 percent between 1979 and 1983 to 6.9 percent between 1984 and 1988), Congress turned its attention to Part B, with an average annual growth rate of nearly 20 percent.[4] The Deficit Reduction Act of 1984 placed a freeze on customary and prevailing charge screens through December 31, 1986, and created a participating physician program. Under this program, physicians could, as previously, opt on a case-by-case basis whether (1) to bill Medicare directly and thereby accept Medicare reimbursement as payment in full ("accept assignment") or (2) to bill the patient for the full charges, with the patient collecting from Medicare. However, those who contracted to accept assignment on all claims for service to Medicare patients during the contract year were granted certain advantages as participating providers: listings in widely distributed directories and, theoretically, expedited bill processing, in addition to reduction of the bad debt problem. Furthermore, the fee freeze for participating physicians was lifted eight months before that for nonparticipating physicians, with a 4 percent increase in prevailing fees.

This prevailing fee screen differential between participating and nonparticipating physicians has since been retained with subsequent increases in fee screens. Moreover, nonparticipating physicians, who saw not only fee screens, but also actual charges frozen during the fee freeze, have since that time been subjected to a complicated maximum allowable actual charge limit.[3,5] The disadvantages of nonparticipation had by the end of 1988 induced over 37 percent of physicians to sign participation agreements, up from 30 percent in the previous years; the assignment rate for physician services (including assignment for nonparticipating physician services) reached 78 percent at the and of 1988.[6]

Another limitation recently applied to Part B reimbursement in an attempt to control costs is the concept of inherent reasonableness of charges. The 1986 and 1987 Omnibus Budget Reconciliation Acts explicitly authorize Medicare and its carriers to modify existing CPR rates to reflect inherent reasonableness, taking into account such criteria as the costs of providing a service and the technological changes not reflected in charges. Pursuant to the congressional mandate set forth in this legislation, DHHS undertook a review of payment for fourteen of the most costly procedures under Part B, such as cataract removal, coronary artery bypass, and total hip replacement. Finding these procedures overvalued, it directed a reduction in charges, starting with cataract surgery in 1988. By restricting the actual charges for nonparticipating physicians performing these procedures, the 1986 legislation also attempted to limit the extent to which physicians can offset reductions in Medicare payments by increasing charges to beneficiaries.

This increasingly complex patchwork of accumulated fee constraints has resulted in a reimbursement structure that is administratively cumbersome and, in the eyes of many practitioners, arcane and unpredictable. Furthermore, the increasing fee squeeze has highlighted biases built into Medicare's CPR payment system. As adopted in 1965 from existing private insurance models that provided fairly comprehensive coverage of inpatient but not outpatient care, the CPR system generally favors inpatient, procedure-oriented, urban-based subspecialty care. It has been criticized for "encouraging physicians to specialize, to practice in urban and suburban areas, and to perform services in hospital settings—all in the face of stated national policies of encouraging primary care, rural practice and out-of-hospital services."[7] The result has been increasing pressure for reform of the existing payment system.

MEDICARE REIMBURSEMENT: REFORM INITIATIVES

Resource-Based Relative-Value Scales

It is against this background that the 1985 Budget Reconciliation Act mandated that DHHS construct a resource-based relative-value scale (RBRVS) for physician services and advise Congress by 1990 on the feasibility of formulating a more rational, RBRVS-based indemnity fee schedule to replace the old CPR system. To undertake the RBRVS analysis, the Health Care Financing Administration (HCFA), the DHHS agency that administers Medicare, contracted with a team of researchers at the Harvard School of Public Health headed by William C. Hsiao, an economics professor.

Concluding a three-year research effort, the Hsiao team published its long-awaited study in September 1988.[8] The study constructs a relative-value scale for physician services based on resource inputs, including (1) total work input performed by the physician for each service, (2) practice costs, including malpractice premiums; and (3) the cost of specialty training. The most subjective of these measurements, total work input, was evaluated by time spent before, during, and after the particular service and by the intensity with which that time is spent. This latter criterion was further broken down into the following dimensions: (1) time, (2) mental effort and judgment, (3) technical skill, and (4) psychological stress. The study drew on highly consistent and reproducible relative-work ratings by surveyed physicians for particular services in their specialty. Using this method, a ratio scale was set up for services in each specialty in relation to a reference service—for example, uncomplicated inguinal hernia repair for the specialty of General Surgery. In order to create a common scale for all the specialties, linkages were established with the help of the cross-specialty physician advisory panel by identifying pairs of services from different specialties that required approximately equal amounts of work. In this manner, RBRVS

Figure 12.1
**Results of a Simulation of the Impact of an RBRVS-Based Fee Schedule on 1986
Medicare Payments, According to Specialty**

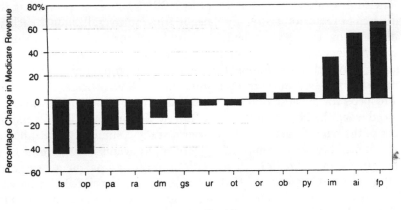

Total Medicare payments in each specialty were calculated from the RBRVS, service volume,
and a monetary conversion factor. **ts** denotes thoracic and cardiovascular surgery, **op** ophthalmology, **pa** pathology, **ra** radiology, **dm** dermatology, **gs** general surgery, **ur** urology, **ot**
otolaryngology, **or** orthopedic surgery, **ob** obstetrics and gynecology, **py** psychiatry, **im** internal
medicine, **ai** allergy and immunology, and **fp** family practice. (Reproduced with permission of
New England Journal of Medicine 319 (1988): 881–88.)

figures were developed for some 2,000 services coded in the insurance carriers' reference, *Physicians' Current Procedural Terminology* (CPT–4), accounting for 80 percent of Medicare payments to physicians in fourteen
specialties.

Evaluating current Medicare charges in the light of RBRVS, the study
found that, in general, evaluation and management services (whether by
internists, surgeons, or other specialists) are compensated at less than half
the rate of invasive, imaging, and laboratory services relative to resource
input, with the gap widest for outpatient cognitive services. Certain invasive
procedures were found to be compensated at rates far out of proportion to
resource input. For example, a colonoscopy at a surgery center, requiring
about five times more resources than a general intermediate-length office
visit, was compensated by Medicare in 1986 at a rate twenty-five times
higher than the office visit. Similarly, triple-vessel coronary artery bypass
surgery, requiring 30 times more resources than an intermediate office visit,
was compensated at a rate 160 times higher.

Assuming constant total Medicare payments to physicians, the study estimated that adoption of an RBRVS-based fee schedule could result in significant changes in Medicare payment patterns for various specialties, as
illustrated in Figure 12.1.[9] For example, an average family practitioner could

receive 60 to 70 percent more in revenues from Medicare. By contrast, the average ophthalmologist and thoracic and cardiovascular surgeon could receive 40 to 50 percent less in revenues from Medicare.

The study evaluated the validity of its RBRVS figures by comparing them with fees in Ontario. There, after negotiating an overall budget each year with the provincial government, the provincial medical society brings together representatives of the major specialties to negotiate a uniform and equitable fee schedule among themselves. The study found the ratio of Ontario fees to be similar to that under the RBRVS scheme.

Prospects for the adoption of a fee schedule based on an RBRVS were enhanced when the Physician Payment Review Commission (PPRC) endorsed most of the basic findings of the Harvard study.[6] The PPRC, an influential thirteen-member board composed largely of physicians and economists, was set up by Congress in 1985 to advise it on physician payment issues. In its 1989 *Report to Congress*, the PPRC recommended that an RBRVS-based national Medicare fee schedule covering all specialties be phased in over a two-year period, replacing the current charge-based reimbursement system.

The PPRC recommendation incorporates the work component of the RBRVS essentially as derived by the Harvard study, although it drops the training cost component and changes the calculation of practice costs in a way that could nearly halve payment shifts projected under the Hsiao formula. Under the PPRC proposal, uniform global fees for surgical procedures would replace the pre-, intra-, and postservice packages devised by Hsiao. Evaluation and management visit codes would be modified to incorporate time as well as site, patient type, and referral status. In addition, a geographic multiplier would be permitted to adjust fees for regional variations in cost.

Intense lobbying by various specialty groups standing to gain or lose from the RBRVS began immediately after publication of the Hsiao study and is likely to affect the ultimate outcome. The director of the American College of Surgeons (ACS), for example, expressed "strenuous opposition," while the American Society of Internal Medicine warmly praised the study.[10] Even before the final RBRVS findings were released, the American College of Radiology, anticipating "loser" status under the RBRVS, sought to preempt the Harvard study by negotiating its own fee schedule with Congress. More recently, the ACS has similarly attempted to pre-empt a cross-specialty, RBRVS-based fee schedule by proposing to Congress its own separately negotiated fee schedule, based more heavily on historical charges than on resources.

What effect, if any, adoption of an RBRVS-based fee schedule would per se have on overall Medicare Part B costs is unclear. As discussed below, many state Medicaid programs shifted in the 1970s from CPR reimbursement to some form of fee schedule as a means of containing payments; however, in view of the already extensive regulatory constraints in the current Medicare CPR reimbursement system, it is questionable whether adoption of a fee-schedule approach would of itself significantly contribute to cost containment at this point. The Hsiao study argues that a fee schedule based on the RBRVS might encourage a shift away from expensive, invasive, hospital-based procedures and diagnostic tests and, as a result, lower the cost of medical care. On the other hand, saving from reduced use of these services might be offset by increased expenditures on services with increased relative values. Furthermore, some physicians might offset decreases in payment rates by increasing the volume and intensity of these service, as to some extent occurred during the 1984–1986 fee freeze. As Dr. William Roper, head of HCFA, noted: "A fee schedule based on RBRVS is designed to reduce perceived inequities in payment and establish fairer relative prices—a goal I support. . . . However, the critical problems of increasing volume and intensity would remain, as they would under any fee for service system."[11]

Moreover, in addition to concerns that an RBRVS would not of itself contain growth in the volume and intensity of physician services, fears have been raised that reduced physician Medicare reimbursement in certain specialties might lead to a decline in the proportion of physicians accepting Medicare assignments and either increased balance billing or decreased access for Medicare beneficiaries. The developing physician surplus in many specialties, in conjunction with the high proportion of the patient population represented by Medicare recipients, may mitigate somewhat the problem of denial of access to Medicare patients, although this could become an issue if rates are set very low, as with Medicaid. However, increased balance billing to offset reductions in Medicare fees is a very real possibility.

To address this problem, some within the Congress and HHS have advocated adoption along with the RBRVS-based fee schedule of a mandatory assignment policy along the lines of the policy recently adopted in Massachusetts. There, physicians are as a condition of licensure obligated to accept assignment as payment in full for services to Medicare patients; balance billing has likewise been prohibited by Massachusetts Blue Shield, which dominates the private insurance market in that state. The Massachusetts law has survived challenges in the lower federal courts by the Massachusetts Medical Society, but remains highly controversial and strongly opposed by physician groups.

At the federal level since the 1985 Budget Reconciliation Act the fee-schedule payment with mandatory assignment has been the rule under Medicare for ambulatory laboratory services, including those in physicians' offices. For the time being, HCFA and PPRC have largely refrained from advocating the extension of mandatory assignment to payment for physician services. However, along with its recommendations for an RBRVS-based fee schedule, the 1989 PPRC *Report to Congress* would eliminate balance billing for certain low-income beneficiaries whose Medicare premiums and coinsurance are paid by state Medicaid programs. It would also limit charges

for unassigned claims to some fixed percentage, such as 125 percent of the
fee-schedule amount.

To address the problem of possible continued fee-for-service incentives
to increase the volume and intensity of services under an RBRVS-based fee
schedule, HCFA and PPRC are exploring various additional changes in
Medicare reimbursement. One concept being examined is a Canadian-style
budgetary cap on total Part B expenditures, with reimbursement rates within
this budget negotiated by HCFA and physician groups with reference to the
RBRVS. This is, in fact, the approach recommended by the PPRC in its
1989 report; the dollar conversion factor used to convert the relative-value
scale into a national fee schedule would be set each year to meet the annual
Part B national expenditure target.

Another approach being advocated by PPRC to control volume of services
is the development of clinical practice guidelines or protocols for the treatment of particular conditions. Along the same lines, HCFA is undertaking
a review of various expensive, high-volume procedures such as percutaneous
transluminal coronary angioplasty and carotid endarterectomy to determine
indications that are well supported in the medical literature. The implication
of both these approaches is that treatments falling outside of both prescribed
guidelines would be denied reimbursement, as has recently occurred with
the use of the thrombolytic TPA for myocardial infarctions.

Prospective Payment Mechanisms

Although currently somewhat overshadowed by the RBRVS debate, much
of the interest over the past decade in restructuring the Medicare reimbursement system to contain costs has focused on the development of prospective payment mechanisms. One such approach, drawing on the success
of DRGs in restraining Medicare Part A expenditures, would adopt an
analogous system of prospectively determined physician payments under
Part B according to diagnostic category. Most proposals to date have focused
on application of physician DRGs to inpatient services. Under various forms
of these proposals, payment for inpatient services by physicians would be
incorporated into hospital DRGs or paid separately in a lump sum to the
attending physician or hospital staff for allocation among the inpatient
physicians providing services.

However, strong objections to physician DRGs have been raised on the
basis of loss of physician autonomy, physician assumption of unacceptable
risk, and greater administrative complexity compared to hospital DRGs.
These problems, combined with the much larger case volume and variability
involved, would make application of physician DRGs to outpatient practice
even more difficult. In its fiscal 1988 budget proposals, the Reagan administration put forward its first limited physician DRG proposals, which would
have incorporated payments to radiologists, anesthesiologists, and pathol-

ogists into Medicare's DRG payments to hospitals. However, as indicated above, the American College of Radiology managed in congressional hearings to negotiate a separate fee schedule in preference to the DRG approach, and no action was taken on the administration's proposal.

Another prospective reimbursement mechanism explored by Medicare, capitated payments to health maintenance organizations (HMOs), has met with more acceptance. Since early 1985, Medicare beneficiaries have had the option of obtaining care through prepaid plans that have entered into capitation contracts with HCFA. Nearly 1 million beneficiaries have taken advantage of that option, enrolling in one of the 175 prepaid plans contracting with the HCFA. Over half of the participating plans are individual practice association (IPA) model HMOs, the remainder being a mixture of staff/network-model HMOs and prepaid group medical practices. Under these contracts the plan agrees to provide the full package of Medicare-covered services in return for an annual capitation rate set at 95 percent of Medicare's adjusted average per capita cost (AAPCC) for traditional care in the area. The AAPCC is calculated from tables of the average per-beneficiary cost for Medicare Part A and fee-for-service Part B care in the HMO's county of operation, with adjustments for the age, sex, institutional status, and welfare status of the HMO's particular mix of enrollees. However, the HMO is required to plough back to enrollees in the form of increased benefits or decreased premiums any difference between the capitated prepayment and the HMO's costs (as gauged by a calculated "adjusted community rate," including profit margin).[12]

Despite the limitation on profit retention (but not risk exposure) inherent in this arrangement, there has been considerable interest in Medicare contracting in the managed care industry, as the above enrollment figures indicate. HCFA head William Roper and others in the Reagan administration saw Medicare contracting with prepaid plans as a more palatable and cost-effective alternative to more direct forms of fee regulation for controlling Medicare costs. They envisioned a system in which the primary form of provider reimbursement is prospective, in the form of capitated payments to managed care plans selected by Medicare beneficiaries, possibly under a voucher scheme.[13]

However, the enthusiasm for prepaid care among beneficiaries and congressional leaders has, at least in the short run, been dampened somewhat by the recent collapse of Medicare's largest HMO contract, with Florida's International Medical Centers (IMC), amidst charges of profiteering by screening out high-risk enrollees, providing substandard care, and engaging in questionable financial practices. In the wake of the IMC debacle, the HCFA and Congress have examined the need for closer monitoring of Medicare-HMO contracts and have adopted HMO peer review requirements and prohibitions against HMO incentive payments to physicians for reducing services to beneficiaries. At the same time, as capitated payments lag, pegged to constrained Medicare fee-for-service rates, a few well-respected HMO contractors in certain areas have recently withdrawn from Medicare participation.

In sum, movement in the direction of prospective payment, favored by many in government, has been halting. Arrangements such as managed care contracts may come to play a more important role over the longer run as government cost containment efforts intensify. However, in the immediate future, less radical departures from the current system can be expected, such as adoption of some form of RBRVS-based fee schedule.

PHYSICIAN REIMBURSEMENT UNDER MEDICAID

Medicaid, the major government program providing health care coverage for the indigent, was enacted by Congress as Title XIX of the Social Security Act in 1965, shortly after the passage of Medicare. Under Title XIX, federal funds were made available to states for comprehensive health care programs covering recipients of federal categorical public assistance grants [mainly Aid to Families with Dependent Children (AFDC) and Social Security Insurance (SSI)], as well as other state-designated medically indigent persons. These matching federal funds pay from 50 to 83 percent of the costs of the state Medicaid programs, depending on state per capita income.

Title XIX generally left administration of the Medicaid program to the states, including determination of provider reimbursement. For ease of administration and encouragement of physician participation, most state Medicaid programs initially adopted Medicare's CPR standard for physician reimbursement. However, under increased pressures to contain Medicaid costs in the 1970s, states that retained this reimbursement method began applying prevailing fee screens substantially more restrictive than Medicare's. By the early 1980s two-thirds of the states had changed to fee schedules, which generally set low rates of reimbursement and were only infrequently updated. In most states the ratio of Medicaid to Medicare fee levels continued to drop through the mid-1980s; in some states, such as New York and Pennsylvania, this ratio was less than 25 percent, leading to physician complaints that Medicaid reimbursement did not even cover their overhead expenses. Paralleling these trends in physician reimbursement has been a sharp decline in physician participation in Medicaid and increasing reliance by the Medicaid population on the expensive alternative of hospital emergency rooms and outpatient departments.

Confronted with the problem of providing more cost-effective care, many state Medicaid programs have, like Medicare, shown increasing interest in prospective methods of provider reimbursement. Analogous to the Medicare system, DRG-based systems of hospital reimbursement have been widely adopted. Some twenty states have, in addition, developed primary care case management programs; almost half of these involve some form of capitated prepayments for primary care and referral services, along the lines of an HMO or a preferred provider organization (PPO). In Arizona and several other states, contracts setting prospective payments for both impatient and outpatient services have been awarded on the basis of competitive bidding. Through state programs of this sort, nearly 1 million Medicaid recipients have been enrolled in HMOs or similar prepaid plans. Data are not yet available on how successful these programs have, in fact, been in providing cost-effective care to Medicaid patients. As with Medicare, the prospects for continued long-term growth of programs of this sort are likely to depend on the capitation rates required to attract provider participation; quality control measures will also be important to prevent repetition of the sorts of abuses that ended California's initial experiment with HMO Medicaid enrollment in the early 1970s.

UNCLEAR PROSPECTS

There has been increasing dissatisfaction among both payers and providers with Medicare's CPR reimbursement system, as modified by a patchwork of fee constraints and regulations. In the short run, limited reform of this system, as through the adoption of an RBRVS-based fee schedule, is likely. The prospects over the longer run for more far-reaching changes, such as capitated programs, remain unclear at this time. The payment structure finally adopted by Medicare is likely to strongly influence both Medicaid and private third-party payers.

NOTES

1. Health Care Financing Administration, *Health Care Financing Review* 8:1 (1986): 17.
2. Social Security Amendments of 1965, P.L. 89–97, Section 1842; Part B, XVIII.
3. See the discussion in P. R. Lee and P. B. Ginsburg, "Building a Consensus for Physician Payment Reform in Medicare," *Western Journal of Medicine* 149:3 (1988): 352–58.
4. J. K. Inglehart, "Payment of Physicians Under Medicare," *New England Journal of Medicine* 318 (1988): 863–69.
5. See also American College of Physicians, Health and Public Policy Committee, "Medicare Payment for Physician Services," *Annals of Internal Medicine* 106:1 (1987): 151–63.
6. Physician Payment Review Commission, *Annual Report to Congress* (Washington, D.C.: Physician Payment Review Commission, 1989).
7. S. F. Jencks and A. Dobson, "Strategies for Reforming Medicare's Physician Payments: Physician Diagnosis Related Groups and Other Approaches," *New England Journal of Medicine* 312 (1985): 1492–99.
8. W. C. Hsiao et al., "Results and Policy Implication of the Resource-Based Relative-Value Study," *New England Journal of Medicine* 319:13 (1988): 881–88.

9. Ibid., p. 886.

10. R. Spence, "New Fee Structure Proposed by Medicare," *Washington Post*, September 29, 1988, p. A3.

11. W. L. Roper, "Perspectives on Physician Payment Reform: The Resource-Based Relative Value Scale in Context," *New England Journal of Medicine* 319:13 (1988): 865–67.

12. J. K. Inglehart, "Second Thoughts About HMOs for Medicare Patients," *New England Journal of Medicine* (1987): 1487–92.

13. J. B. Bautz and T. Wetle, "HMO Enrollment of Medicare Recipients: An Analysis of Incentives and Barriers," *Journal of Health Politics, Policy and Law* (1984): 41–62.

13

The Origins and Consequences of Medicare

Edward Berkowitz and Wendy Wolff

The United States, unlike most European countries, has an ambivalent attitude toward government involvement in paying for medical care. In this country we have decided to use government money to subsidize private practice, rather than giving government the power to organize the delivery and maintain the quality of medical care. American doctors do not work for the government, even though the federal government has become the largest single payer in the health care system.

In an effort to explain the disparity between federal money and federal control, this chapter traces public and private approaches to helping Americans pay their health care bills, from early prepayment and health insurance plans starting in the 1930s to the passage of Medicare and beyond. This chapter takes an explicitly historical approach to its subject in the hope of discovering how old solutions have become transformed into new problems.

COOPERATION AND CONFRONTATION, 1933–1946

In the twentieth century there has been a fundamental tension in health care policy. On the one hand, physicians have taken an entrepreneurial (or artisan's) view of their profession that has sanctified the fee-for-service system and the doctor-patient relationship. Any proposed system of financing medical care that threatens this approach has had to be adapted to the concerns of the medical profession. On the other hand, there has been a recognition that individuals are often unable to bear the costs of their medical treatment and that all citizens should have access to adequate care.

In the 1930s, which might be considered the beginning of the modern era in the doctor/hospital–federal government relationship, national health insurance and private group medical prepayment plans emerged as two prominent proposals to help individuals pay the costs of health care. The idea for a national system of health insurance, which originated in the Progressive era of the early 1900s in a form that was to be implemented by the states, reached its full development in the Depression. During the Progressive era the object was to replace the income foregone by someone who was ill. By the 1930s the goals shifted to payment of hospital fees and doctors' fees.

The staff of the Committee on Economic Security, federal employees who did the background research for the 1935 Social Security Act, prepared an early statement on national health insurance. Ill health posed a grave economic risk, their report suggested, but that risk could be controlled by pooling the costs of ill health across many individuals. The committee staff referred to this notion as group budgeting, which it defined as "budgeting the expenditures so that each family carries an average rather than an uncertain risk."[1]

Considered in this manner, the achievement of national health insurance seemed an easy matter, but in this case, as in many others over the course of the next fifty years, simple academic theories yielded to complex political realities. National health insurance was transformed from a group budgeting program, which could be implemented in isolation from other programs and required no new federal funds, into a complex social insurance scheme that was designed to mesh with the old-age insurance and unemployment compensation programs created by the 1935 Social Security Act. The politics of national health insurance became subsumed in the politics of social security. Difficulties in raising social security benefits and extending social security coverage created problems for national health insurance as well. Political stalemate in one area precluded progress in the other.

If the government failed to achieve group budgeting for health care, the private sector nonetheless produced its own innovations, including early versions of the modern health maintenance organization (HMO). One version originated with Edward A. Filene, the Boston department store owner who had become interested in social reform.[2] Filene believed that ill health could be largely prevented through a system of comprehensive health care financed on a prepayment basis, which he likened to preventive maintenance, "much as an engineer would give to his machine."[3] Even when the issue of federal intervention in the health care market became more pressing during the Depression, Filene clung to a Progressive era belief that the government's proper role lay in mobilizing the private sector, rather than in acting on its own. He therefore encouraged action by the Twentieth Century Fund, a private foundation for which Filene provided most of the support, in the field of medical economics. In particular, Filene and his assistants tried to spark interest among private agencies in what they called "prepaid group health plans."[4] By this, they meant plans that would bring together a comprehensive group of medical specialists who would supply a wide range of medical services, including hospitalization, for a predetermined fee.

In 1937 the employees of the Home Owners Loan Corporation (HOLC) formed a nonprofit corporation to furnish medical care to themselves and their families. The HOLC was a government agency, but its employees acted as private individuals in establishing the nonprofit corporation, which they named the Group Health Association (GHA). GHA employed its own staff of salaried physicians who provided care in a downtown Washington, D.C., medical center that GHA owned and operated. Today, the arrangement would be called a staff-model HMO.

GHA's founding provided an early test of whether physicians would agree to depart from a fee-for-service arrangement and become employees of prepaid health plans. The local medical community reacted warily, fearing that GHA would rake off the paying patients and leave the medically indigent to the rest of the doctors. Since the indigent patients already received discounts, some doctors believed GHA would bankrupt local physicians and seriously undermine the quality of medical care in the Washington, D.C., area.

Because of these fears, the Medical Society of the District of Columbia launched a campaign to hinder the functioning of GHA. The society forbade its members to work for the organization, threatening any physician employed by GHA with expulsion and withdrawal of privileges to practice in local hospitals. Further, the society and the American Medical Association (AMA) attacked the legal basis of GHA, questioning its right to practice medicine as a corporation. The society also enlisted the aid of local hospitals, insisting that they should permit only members of the local medical society to serve on their staffs. Since GHA physicians were refused membership in the medical society, they would thus be barred from the hospitals. The hospitals, for their part, treated GHA as if it did not exist, refusing even to cash GHA checks. The first modern HMO, in other words, met with an extremely hostile reception from doctors who wished to preserve the fee-for-service system.

GHA soon emerged as a major political issue, one of the first confrontations between the federal government and the AMA. Government officials realized that the failure of GHA would represent a significant defeat for the principle of prepaid group health care. Accordingly, the Roosevelt administration, acting through the Department of Justice, launched a rescue mission. In July 1938 Thurman Arnold, who headed the Justice Department's Antitrust Division, formally charged the AMA and the Medical Society of the District of Columbia with violating the antitrust laws of the United States. In December 1938 a grand jury indicted the AMA and the medical society for violating the Sherman Antitrust Act.

After lengthy legal delays, the case finally came to trial in 1941, and extensive testimony about the medical society's campaign against GHA was

offered. The defense attorneys tried to make socialized medicine and professional control of medicine the issues in the trial, but the jury found the
AMA and the local medical society guilty, a verdict that was upheld by a
unanimous Supreme Court in January 1943.

The case indicated the lengths to which the government was prepared to
go in an effort to establish prepaid group health plans with salaried physicians. As a practical matter, the tool of antitrust litigation was a crude
one, but it had the potential advantage of bypassing a stalemated Congress
and intervening directly in medical practice at the local level. On the one
hand, the reassuring and traditional approach of prosecution under the
antitrust laws masked the radical nature of the government's intentions. It
reduced the effort to establish staff-model HMOs to a matter of economic
freedom, in which the government acted on the consumer's behalf. On the
other hand, using the case-by-case approach through the legal system was
a painfully slow way to remedy social problems.

By the time the GHA case was decided in 1943 the federal government
had retreated from its strong advocacy of prepaid group health plans. With
prosperity during wartime, more people could afford to pay for health care
on a traditional fee-for-service basis. The government discreetly backed
away from prepaid group practice as a policy goal and instead relied on
more indirect forms of aid to the health care system. Rather than challenging
the terms of doctors' employment, the government helped to finance the
infrastructure that supported modern medical care.

VOLUNTARY HEALTH INSURANCE AND GOVERNMENT
AID TO HOSPITALS, 1946–1950

Group budgeting caught on in the postwar era, and third-party payment
came to dominate the market for medical care. The use of health insurance
grew dramatically, and by 1951 over 40 million Americans were covered
by private health insurance plans, often with the financial assistance of the
breadwinner's employer. In that same year 37.4 million Americans received
the benefits of a hospital "assurance" plan, known as Blue Cross, which
paid hospital bills in return for the receipt of a level monthly fee. Only 1.4
million people belonged to a Blue Cross plan in 1938 (Law, 1974, p. 11).

The new health care financing system centered on the hospital. People
correctly perceived that hospital stays, rather than routine visits to the
doctors, imposed unpredictable and often catastrophic costs on family budgets. Assisted by the hospitals and the private insurance companies, such
as Aetna and Prudential, cautious consumers allowed their employers to
purchase group insurance plans that spread the risks over large groups and
reduced average health care costs. Most employees then shared the costs of
this group insurance with their employers, often with the administrative
assistance of trade unions. The system handled the costs of both hospital

care and physicians' services that were incurred during hospital stays, such as the surgeon's fee for performing an operation and the radiologist's fee for reading an x-ray. Although a private insurance company now reimbursed the individual for physicians' fees, the doctors continued to work on a fee-for-service basis. Routine care, such as an annual checkup or a well baby's visit to a pediatrician, remained unreimbursed. Although HMOs existed in various pockets of the country—such as Washington, D.C.; Oakland; Seattle; and Minneapolis—they stood on the fringes of medical practice. Americans had opted, in effect, for budgeting catastrophic health care costs across many private groups and preserving the physician's right to bill on a fee-for-service basis.

The postwar medical care system also permitted a role for the federal government. The provision of care was a private matter; however, the construction of hospitals and the support of private research were matters of public finance. In 1946, for example, Congress passed the Hospital Survey and Construction Act, better known as the Hill-Burton Act for its chief sponsors, Democratic Senator Lister Hill of Alabama and Republican Representative Harold Burton of Ohio. Efforts to pass this law brought together a wide coalition of political interests, ranging from the U.S. Chamber of Commerce and the American Medical Association on the right to the labor unions and the social security bureaucracy on the left. The resulting law provided federal funds for building local hospitals.[5]

Conferring federal largess on the hospital, rather than on the doctors who practiced there, proved to be a shrewd political choice. For one thing, hospitals, unlike, say, facilities for the mentally ill, were a politically popular cause. Their popularity reflected the transformation of the hospital that was nearly complete by the end of World War II. In the middle of the nineteenth century the hospital was a welfare institution, like a prison or an insane asylum, that attracted transients and other marginal members of society. Others received their care at home. In the twentieth century, however, hospitals escaped from their asylum origins and middle-class people started to use them. By 1920 private paying patients outnumbered the charity cases, and, as a consequence, more than half of the hospitals' income came from private patients. As hospitals grew in stature, creating more of them became a national priority.[6]

For another thing, hospital construction produced fewer political problems than did proposals that involved the government in the more intimate details of patient care. The Hill-Burton Act observed the political proprieties. It allowed maximum discretion to hospital administrators (who were to approve state hospital construction plans) and to local governments. Because the act was also compatible with a health-planning approach to the construction of health facilities, it experienced few political difficulties at a time when national health insurance was contested along deep partisan lines.

Much the same could be said of government aid for the conduct of medical research. It also allowed private doctors to control the use of federal funds. One popular strategy that began in earnest in 1946 was for doctors in a particular specialty to request the formation of a National Institute of Health. This institute would then award research and other grants to medical scientists, often doctors affiliated with medical schools. Physicians in such settings worked on salary far more often than did their counterparts in private practice, and nearly all of these "research" doctors came to depend on government grants to support themselves and their laboratories. These physicians, more removed from routine clinical practice than were their private practice peers, tolerated this government intrusion in part because it occurred on such permissive terms. The government did not presume to influence the course of private research or medical care; instead, it sought to direct public funds to the researchers who, in the opinion of their medical school colleagues, showed scientific promise. Once again, it was a matter of private control over public money that had the ultimate effect of improving the quality of medical practice.

TOWARD MEDICARE AND MEDICAID

The only problem with this postwar system of financing health care was that it still left gaps in coverage or access. As sociologist Paul Starr has noted, the system did little to help the "poor, for whom health insurance was originally conceived" (Starr, 1982, p. 289). It also squeezed people who were not natural members of an employer-based group, such as the elderly. Because many older people were no longer working, they were forced to purchase individual, rather than group, policies. Some of the elderly—just how many is difficult to estimate—consequently faced prohibitive costs for health insurance and ended up depleting their resources during a spell of illness. In the postwar era the federal government did much to close these gaps in the system while, at the same time, preserving the system's basic character.

The first significant government intervention involved assuring health care to those on welfare. In 1950 the federal government allowed state and local governments to make payments to local medical vendors who supplied welfare recipients with medical care. Then, in 1960, the government took a second step and created a program of federal grants to the states and localities to pay for medical care to the elderly on welfare or to the elderly who were "medically indigent."

This second measure came to be associated with the congressional sponsors of the legislation, Oklahoma Democratic Senator Robert S. Kerr and Arkansas Democratic Representative Wilbur D. Mills. The Kerr-Mills approach proved to be less than a total success. Indirect and permissive aid worked well for hospital construction and the support of research; it functioned less effectively when the issue was access to care. Kerr-Mills yielded widely different forms of care from state to state, appearing to discriminate against the elderly on the basis of locality. Thus, New Jersey, which passed a Kerr-Mills program that was administered by the local Blue Cross–Blue Shield plan, allowed 365 inpatient days a year; Wyoming, with a program also administered by Blue Cross–Blue Shield, permitted only 70 inpatient days a year.[7] As late as 1963, Kerr-Mills programs existed in only thirty-six states.[8]

In the late 1950s there occurred a resurgence of interest in national health insurance that would include all the elderly, rather than just the elderly receiving welfare. The distinction between the national health insurance (or Medicare) and the Kerr-Mills approaches resembled that between social security and welfare. Social security went to all workers who had paid social security taxes, which meant nearly all the workers in the labor force, while only those who could demonstrate that they were poor received welfare. The campaign in the 1950s involved the provision of health insurance for all social security beneficiaries. Unlike earlier health insurance campaigns, then, this one excluded Americans of working age who, presumably, were provided for by the existing system.

Although the government had, in effect, conceded working Americans to the private health insurance industry, the new campaign for health insurance under the banner of Medicare generated its share of political controversy. Liberals wanted the federal government to pay for the hospital care of the elderly; conservatives believed that such legislation would be the means through which the federal government crossed the threshold of financial support and came to control the provision of medical care. The fear expressed by the AMA was that health insurance for the elderly, such as Medicare, would finally allow the federal government to set physicians' salaries and regulate working conditions. Far better, the AMA believed, to restrict government subsidies to the poor and to administer such programs at the local level. Far better, the liberals countered, to utilize the tried and trusted social security system and provide federally administered health insurance that would not involve the stigma of welfare.

The AMA wielded considerable political power in the deliberations preceding the passage of Medicare. It took the death of a president and substantial concessions on the part of federal administrators to produce legislation in 1965. Because of the many interests accommodated by the legislation, Medicare emerged as a very complex law. Despite this complexity, it did little to alter the existing system of paying the physician. In the short run, at least, few of the AMA's fears were realized.

The law contained three major parts. Part A of Medicare permitted the elderly to receive health insurance at no cost, except for the copayments and deductibles that were typical of private health insurance. This part of the law depended on financial contributions from the social security taxes of the working population. It applied only to hospital care, and not to

physician-provided care. Doctors, at least in theory, did not receive reimbursement through Part A.

Hospitals, however, managed quite well under Part A's provisions. Instead
of receiving an agreed-on rate, the hospitals were allowed to bill the government on the "reasonable cost basis" that was customary under Blue
Cross.[9] Congress became quite explicit on the subject of allowable costs.
The Senate Finance Committee noted that since the law would follow the
principle of reasonable cost, "hospitals would not be deterred, because of
nonpaying or underpaying patients in this aged group, from trying to provide
the best of modern care." This same committee mentioned that whatever
specific reimbursement method was used, hospitals should be allowed to
recover both their direct and indirect costs, including depreciation on buildings and equipment, the costs of capital indebtedness, and a portion of the
net costs of educational activities (such as stipends for teachers).[10] Concessions to the hospitals went even further: Hospitals were not required to
deal directly with the federal government, but instead could handle their
financial affairs though a "fiscal intermediary," often a local Blue Cross
plan (Law, 1974, pp. 59–61, 72).

In keeping with the modern politics of health insurance and mindful of
the AMA's power, the administration had wanted to stop at Part A. The
politics of enactment pushed Congress farther, however, and led to Medicare
Part B, designed to handle doctors' bills. Part B originated in a proposal by
Representative John W. Byrnes (R–Wisc.) who urged a voluntary program
of federal health insurance that the elderly would finance themselves. Such
a program would be less intrusive on the health care system than the administration's social security–based proposal.

In the final legislative deliberations, Representative Mills, chairman of the
House Committee on Ways and Means, married the administration and the
Byrnes proposals. Mills wanted to protect the social security funds against
bankruptcy. Hence, he allowed doctors' services to be paid in part from the
elderly's contributions and in part from general revenues, and he limited
social security's liability to hospital bills. The administration got a modified
version of its proposal in Medicare Part A, which paid hospital bills and
required no further contributions from the elderly beyond the copayment
and deductible. Byrnes got a modified version of his proposal in Medicare
Part B, which paid doctors' bills but did not use social security contributions.
Part A was compulsory; Part B was voluntary.

Adding to the complexity of the legislation, Mills also included a separate
program that extended the Kerr-Mills program of 1960. Known as Medicaid, this legislation helped to pay the hospital and doctors' bills of welfare
beneficiaries. Where previously the federal government had subsidized the
medical costs of the elderly on welfare, the Medicaid program applied to
all welfare beneficiaries, including the blind, dependent children and their
families, and the permanently and totally disabled.

The Medicare law resembled other Great Society legislation in that Congress, attempting to satisfy everyone, simultaneously adopted competing proposals. Providers and physicians could point to the generous reimbursement terms. Indeed, just as hospitals were to be paid according to "reasonable costs," so physicians' fees would be based on "reasonable and customary" charges. That provision guaranteed that the doctors would receive at least as much from Medicare as they did from other insurance carriers. The Medicare legislation would not be used to force down doctors' fees.[11]

Fiscal conservatives could point to the ways in which the social security trust funds were protected (because they would not be used to pay doctors' bills). The Social Security Administration, represented by Commissioner Robert Ball, had wanted to include hospital-centered specialty care, such as radiology, pathology, and anesthesiology, in Part A. The AMA preferred to put such doctor-supplied services in Part B, and Wilbur Mills tended to side with the AMA since he wanted to be able to say on the House floor that no physicians' fees were covered by social security. When the Speaker of the House pressed Mills on this point, Mills remained adamant.[12]

Robert Ball and Wilbur Cohen, the primary policy entrepreneurs for the Social Security Administration and the Johnson administration, turned to Democratic Senator Paul Douglas of Illinois and persuaded him to offer an amendment in the Senate to restore the specialist payments in Part A. Douglas' amendment passed, setting up a confrontation in the conference committee. Cohen, noted for his ability to offer reasonable compromises, hoped that the conference committee would split the difference. Radiologists and pathologists could be covered under Part A, anesthesiologists under Part B. Cohen counted the American Hospital Association and the AFL-CIO among his supporters, but Mills, Representative Hale Boggs (D–La.), and Senators Russell Long (D–La.) and George Smathers (D–Fla.), who depended on the support of the AMA, won the battle. Cohen wrote that the "conferees action . . . will make the leaders of the AMA happy and the result will be viewed as defeat for the administration."[13]

Liberals, defeated in the boundary battle over Parts A and B, could still tout the complete nature of the coverage (with hospital and doctors' bills both paid). Some liberals, such as Abraham Ribicoff, a Democratic senator from Connecticut, had worried that passage of hospital insurance alone would lead to a political backlash on the part of the elderly. Too many of the elderly, Ribicoff had urged the president, "believe *all* of their medical bills will be paid, not just the hospital and related charges." Ribicoff had requested that a package of benefits be added "on top of" the administration bill.[14] The final legislation did just that.

Acceptable to so many conflicting interests, the Medicare law represented an incremental change in health care policy, rather than a sharp break with the past. Its benefit formula focused, as in private health insurance, on care that was provided in the hospital, rather than on preventive care or long-term custodial care. The terms of reimbursement allowed the federal government to continue its policy of contributing to hospital construction, medical research, and medical education. The law even permitted both hospitals and doctors to utilize familiar institutions, such as Blue Cross and Blue Shield, in the handling of routine transactions. That meant that the law represented the same sort of passive intervention into the market for health care that the Hill-Burton legislation and other health care programs of the postwar era did.

AFTER MEDICARE

One could argue that the public and private sectors reached a truce in 1965. The federal government paid the medical bills of the elderly, and the private sector provided health insurance coverage for nearly everyone else who was not receiving welfare. The terms of this truce have held. Visions of national health insurance, federally administered and universal in coverage, have faded. The private sector continues to supply health insurance to working Americans, and, if anything, private responsibilities have grown in recent years. Even liberals now envision mandated private coverage, rather than ambitious national health insurance, as the way to solve problems of access.[4]

At the same time, the federal government no longer acts so passively in reimbursing doctors and hospitals for services rendered to the elderly or to welfare recipients. Where once doctors and hospitals sent bills to fiscal intermediaries and the federal government gratefully paid them, now the federal government has begun to question the efficiency of this arrangement. The government's long-latent regulatory potential has begun to be realized.

Until the passage of Medicare, the progressive faith had been that the cost of medical care to the individual payer was too high and that the costs needed to be distributed bettei through group budgeting. After the passage of Medicare, however, the focus shifted from providing access to care to the need to control costs. Total costs were now the problem, leading policy analysts to complain that the nation was spending too much of its income on health care.

Medicare played an important role in the public's perception of the problem. As the largest single payer in a highly balkanized medical care market, Medicare figured prominently in the litany of health care cost inflation. In the five years after Medicare began, the cost of medical services grew by 7.9 percent annually, compared to only 3.2 percent a year in the seven years before Medicare, while the federal share of health expenditures rose from 26 to 37 percent between 1965 and 1970. By 1978, analysts have noted, public programs underwrote nearly 90 percent of hospital expenditures made for care of the elderly (Starr, 1982, p. 384; Achenbaum, 1986, p. 172).

Increases both in the cost of health care and in the cost of Medicare were hardly surprising. By making health care accessible to nearly all the elderly, Medicare increased the demand for health care and, in so doing, raised the price. Medicare itself contained few protections against rising costs. Instead, the program allowed providers to pass costs along to the government.

In the long run, as prices continued to rise, both parts of Medicare faced problems. The social security trust funds that financed Part A were not unlimited. In the first place, the relationship between contributions and expenditures was vague since the present generation of workers was financing the health care of the present group of retirees. The health care expenditures of the retirees bore no particular relationship to the social security taxes being paid by the workers. Higher costs meant higher taxes, the diversion of money from the old-age or disability trust funds to the Medicare trust fund, or reduced expenditures. Since the old-age and disability trust funds were financially strapped from the mid-seventies to the early eighties, that left only the alternatives of higher taxes or reduced expenditures, neither of which was politically attractive. The result was a search for ways to make the program function more efficiently in an effort to contain costs while preserving access.

Part B ran into similar problems related to costs. Controlling the costs of this part of the program could require spending more general revenues for Medicare at a time when the federal budget was perceived to be in a significant deficit. Another alternative involved raising the premiums that the elderly paid for Part B, which, since these "premiums" were paid as deductions from a retiree's social security check, had the effect of lowering social security benefits. A final alternative was to reduce payments to doctors. As with Part A, none of these alternatives promised much popularity to the politician who lent his support.

As cost became a pressing problem, health care policy came to resemble other forms of social welfare policy. Economists looked for disincentives to the rational consumption of medical care. In the Medicare program, these were not hard to find since the system paid providers to raise costs rather than to lower them.

Searching for a solution, a new generation discovered prepaid group practice and converted it into the terms of the new cost-conscious policy. In 1973, for example, Congress passed the Health Maintenance Organization Act, which encouraged the growth of such prepaid group plans. When Edward A. Filene had urged the formation of the Group Health Association, he wanted to bring medical care within middle-class means. When the Nixon and Carter administrations encouraged the creation of health maintenance organizations (HMOs), they wanted to use prepaid group practice as a form of health promotion, forestalling expensive care, and as a type of hospital broker, limiting the frequency and duration of hospitalization. The key feature of an HMO was prepayment. Payment of a specific sum in advance set a limit on how much the government or employer would have to pay for a person's health care. It therefore put a limit on health care expenditures and encouraged providers to avoid unnecessary laboratory tests and hospitalization. For Edward Filene, prepayment guaranteed consumers access and freed them from catastrophic costs; for Paul Ellwood and the latter-day discoverers of the HMOs, prepayment set limits on health care expenditures and freed society from uncontrollable costs.

Medicare received similar treatment at the hands of the economists. The reformers introduced a system that attempted to cap payments to providers through a device called prospective payment, which meant, simply, advance payment. The government converted Part A of Medicare into a reimbursement scheme that paid hospitals a fixed amount for a particular diagnosis. A patient's treatment would fit into one or more diagnosis-related groups (DRGs). Efficient hospitals, at least in theory, that could deliver care at a cost below that set for the diagnosis-related group stood to reap rewards; inefficient hospitals would be forced to reduce costs or go out of business. The system functioned with the impartiality of the market, acting as a force to drive down costs.

Theory and reality could, however, diverge. Problems with the prospective reimbursement system included the need to maintain the quality of care. It was often difficult to distinguish efficiency from reduced quality since both have the effect of cutting costs. Also, because there was no theoretically correct level of payment for a particular DRG, payments were politically negotiated. Hence, a provider might well be able to defeat the object of the prospective payment system by simply negotiating a higher rate.

The notion that doctors should be paid on a salaried basis, perhaps with a bonus for extra or exemplary work, has gone from anathema in the early days of GHA to a widely accepted practice today. As the volatility of the health care market increases and as the government and private employers continue to squeeze health care costs, the attractiveness of a salaried position in an HMO, an emergency room, or some sort of group practice should increase. The related notion that the government will use its coercive power to influence doctors' salaries has gone from a fear without much basis in 1965 to a virtual certainty today. The era of third-party reimbursement on the doctors' and hospitals' terms is over. In the future we will begin to pay some of the deferred costs of our permissive system, including those imposed by health care financing programs that tolerate inefficient, expensive medical practice.

NOTES

1. The quotations come from Edgar Sydenstricker and I. S. Falk, "Public Provisions Against the Economic Risks Arising Out of Ill Health," Preliminary Reports,

Committee on Economic Security, September 1934 (Records of the Social Security Administration, RG 47, Accession 56A–533, Washington National Records Center, Suitland, Md.).

2. In this account of the Group Health Association we follow E. Berkowitz and W. Wolff (1988) closely.

3. "Memorandum of the Relation of the Twentieth Century Fund and the Committee on the Costs of Medical Care," Twentieth Century Fund Papers, n.d. See also Edward A. Filene to Professor H. H. Moore, November 1926, and Filene to Roscoe Pound, June 8, 1927, Twentieth Century Fund Papers.

4. *Director's Report, 1936–37* (New York: Twentieth Century Fund, 1937), pp. 16–19. This source is located in the New York headquarters of the Twentieth Century Fund.

5. On the Hill-Burton Act, we rely on House Committee on Interstate and Foreign Commerce, *House Report 2519,* 79th Cong., 2d sess., July 13, 1946, reprinted in *U.S. Code Congressional Service* (Chicago: West and Thompson Company, 1947), pp. 1560–61; the best secondary source is [5], pp. 123–31.

6. For a historical sense of the asylum and of efforts to escape from the asylum in the Progressive era (which it could be argued lasted until 1965), see D. Rothman (1971, 1980). For a view of the development of the hospital, see R. Stevens (1982) and M. J. Vogel (1980).

7. "Meeting of the Consultants on Medical Matters," October 3, 4, 1963 (Records of the Social and Rehabilitation Service, RG 363, Accession 74–30, Box 3, Washington National Records Center, Suitland, Md.).

8. "Possible Improvements in Provision of Medical Assistance to Needy Aged Under OAA and MAA," Staff Paper, April 21, 1964 (RG 235, Accession 69A–1793, Box 41, File AW–5, 1964); Bureau of Family Services, "Minutes of the Meeting of the Consultants on Medical Matters," April 12–13, 1962 (RG 363, Accession 74–30); Ellen Winston to Secretary, January 28, 1964 (RG 235, Accession 69A–1793, File AW–5, Box 41) (Washington National Records Center, Suitland, Md.).

9. "Brief Summary of 'Hospital Insurance, Social Security, and Public Assistance Amendments of 1965,' " December 31, 1964 (RG 235, General Counsel Record, Accession 71A–3497, Box 1, File AW, Washington National Records Center, Suitland, Md.).

10. *Senate Report No. 404,* 89th Cong., 1st sess., March 29, 1965, reprinted in *U.S. Code Congressional and Administrative News,* pp. 1976–77.

11. Technically, doctors were to be paid on a charge basis, and charges were to be "reasonable and not higher than the charge applicable, for a comparable service and under comparable circumstances, to the other policyholders and subscribers of the carrier.... In determining reasonable charges the carriers would consider the customary charge for similar services made by the physician." The usual formulation of this notion is "reasonable and customary" charges. *Senate Report No. 404,* 89th Cong., 1st sess., March 29, 1965, reprinted in *U.S. Code Congressional and Administrative News,* p. 1949.

12. Wilbur Cohen to Secretary, February 8, 1965; Cohen to Lawrence O'Brien, March 17, 1965 (both RG 235, Accession 69A–1793, File LL, Box 16, Washington National Records Center, Suitland, Md.).

13. Cohen to Lawrence O'Brien, July 19, 1965; Cohen to O'Brien, July 20, 1965

(both RG 235, Accession 69A–1793, File LL, Box 16, Washington National Records Center, Suitland, Md.).

14. Abraham Ribicoff to President, March 3, 1965 (RG 235, Accession 69A–1793, File LL, Box 16, Washington National Records Center, Suitland, Md.).

REFERENCES

Achenbaum, A. (1986). *Social Security: Vision and Revision*. New York: Cambridge University Press.

Berkowitz, E. and Wolff, W. (1988). *Group Health Association: A Portrait of a Health Maintenance Organization*. Philadelphia: Temple University Press.

Califano, J. (1981). *Governing America*. New York: Simon and Shuster.

Fein, R. (1986). *Medical Care, Medical Costs*. Cambridge, Mass.: Harvard University Press.

Fox. D. M. (1986). *Health Policies, Health Politics: The British and American Experience, 1911–1965*. Princeton, N.J.: Princeton University Press.

Law, Sylvia. (1974). *Blue Cross: What Went Wrong*. New Haven: Yale University Press.

Rosenberg, C.E. (1979). "Inward Vision and Outward Glance: The Shaping of the American Hospital, 1880–1914." In *Bulletin of the History of Medicine 53*, pp. 346–91.

Rothman, D. (1971). *The Discovery of the Asylum: Social Order and Disorder in the New Republic*. Boston: Little Brown and Company.

———. (1980). *Conscience and Convenience: The Asylum and Its Alternatives in Progressive America*. Boston: Little Brown and Company.

Starr, P. (1982). *The Social Transformation of American Medicine*. New York: Basic Books.

Stevens, R. (1982). " 'A Poor Sort of Memory': Voluntary Hospitals and Government Before the Depression." *Milbank Memorial Fund Quarterly 60*, pp. 551–84.

Voegl, M. J. (1980). *The Invention of the Modern Hospital, Boston, 1870–1930*. Chicago: University of Chicago Press.

14

Medicare as a System

L. Gregory Pawlson

Physician reimbursement under Medicare reflects the issues of physician reimbursement in general, with two areas of special emphasis: Most major decisions concerning the Medicare program are made in the public arena, and Medicare is the largest single physician payer.

The imposition of the third-party payer into the relationship between physician and patient has clearly had a major impact on the amounts of payment and the mechanisms by which physicians are reimbursed for their services. In the case of Medicare, this effect is increased by the fact that the program was formulated and has evolved in the political arena of the federal government. The simple transaction of a patient and physician negotiating a payment before or after some direct service seems far removed from the myriad of special interest groups, congressional committees, commissions, agencies of the federal government, and the judicial system that are involved in setting Medicare physician reimbursement policy. As we will see, the result of these competing interests and jurisdictions is a reimbursement system that is a patchwork of principles, rules, and regulations that are at best inconsistent and often in conflict with each other.

There are several readily apparent reasons for the increasing attention that physician reimbursement in the Medicare program is receiving. For providers, Medicare now accounts for over 20 percent of the total reimbursement to physicians in the United States. While not a dominant force, this market share does create special concern among providers about the reimbursement policies of Medicare. The fact that many private insurance carriers follow Medicare reimbursement policies and decisions adds to the impact. The importance of Medicare reimbursement varies markedly between different medical specialties. On the low end are such specialties as psychiatry and pediatrics where Medicare accounts for less than 5 percent of physician reimbursement. At the other extreme are internal medicine and thoracic surgery at over 30 percent.[1] Obviously, depending on the location of the practice, the age of the physician, and the particular procedure, the rate can vary markedly within a given specialty. For example, some obstetricians/gynecologists may do mostly obstetrics and see virtually no Medicare patients; others do gynecologic oncology and see a high proportion of Medicare patients. There are a small percentage of physicians (about 5 percent) such as ophthalmologists who do almost exclusively cataract surgery or geriatricians whose practice income is almost entirely derived from Medicare.

The obvious reason for the concern on the part of the public and the federal government is the continuing rapid rise of Medicare expenditures for physician services. While overall expenditures for medical care in general, and Medicare in particular, have risen at a rate well in excess of general inflation and the gross national product, expenditures from the Supplementary Medical Insurance Trust Fund, better known as Medicare Part B, have been a particular source of concern. Total expenditures in the United States for physician services have been rising consistently at a yearly rate 3 to 4 percent above inflation. In the Medicare program the rate of rise has been in the 10 to 15 percent per year range or at least 4 to 10 percent above inflation.[2] While the number of Medicare beneficiaries has increased more rapidly than the population in general has, the number eligible has accounted for less than one-fourth of the yearly increase beyond general inflation. Increases in physician prices in excess of general inflation have accounted for another twenty to thirty percent of the increase per year. The major factor, however, has been an increase in service volume and intensity (more services per beneficiary and more costly technology) which has accounted for more than half of the Medicare Part B increase over general inflation.[3]

The increasing expenditures for Medicare physician services have been especially notable with the even more rapid accumulation of yearly budget deficits and a $3 trillion federal debt. The majority (75 percent) of funds for Medicare Part B comes from general revenues rather than the social security trust funds (used for Medicare Part A). Thus, expenditures on Medicare physician reimbursement competes with other areas of the federal budget such as defense, highway programs, and the environment that depend on general tax revenues for their financing. It has not escaped the notice of Congress and the administration that physician reimbursement is a large and rapidly growing area of expenditures in the federal budget.

EARLY MEDICARE PHYSICIAN
REIMBURSEMENT POLICIES

In order to better understand the current problems facing physician services under Medicare, it is important to review the origins and development of the program. It is a common misconception that the physician reimbursement system chosen at the inception of Medicare was modeled after a long-accepted and predominant form of reimbursement in the private insurance sector at the time Medicare was enacted.[4] In actuality, in 1965 the system of paying physicians, termed "usual, customary, and reasonable" or UCR, was a relatively recent addition to physician payment methodology, spurred by the rise in wages and fringe benefits after World War II. Under this method of reimbursement the physician is paid whatever is charged, unless that amount is higher than the physician's usual charge (i.e., the average of charges for the previous year), the customary charge (defined by some percentile, usually the ninetieth, of what all physicians in the area charged for the same service), or what the insurer determined to be "reasonable." The most frequent method of physician reimbursement was still self-pay, accounting for over 70 percent of physician fees at the time. Blue Shield plans, which were among the few private insurers that provided coverage for physician services other than surgery, most commonly used a fee schedule. For persons with low incomes, the physicians accepted the fee schedule as payment in full, while balance billing (i.e., charging the patient over and above what the fee schedule paid) was allowed above a certain income. With the postwar increase in income for employees of large manufacturers, many union members began to exceed the income limit and thus experienced significant out-of-pocket expenses. As a result of this, unions began to demand and large industrial employers began to supply more comprehensive coverage for physician services. However, it was not until after the passage of the Medicare program that most Blue Shield plans and other insurers turned to the UCR methodology.

The political climate surrounding the enactment of Medicare, and specifically the provisions regarding physician reimbursement, was one of frustration, caution, and power struggles.[4, 5] The hospital portion (Part A) of the Medicare program had its origin in the national health insurance proposals of the 1930s and 1940s. Those who advocated national health insurance had been frustrated repeatedly in their effort to enact a program and formulated Medicare as a first step toward their goal. Even this step had been impossible until the Johnson landslide of 1964 and the accompanying demise of the bloc of conservative southern Democrats and Republicans on the House Ways and Means Committee (which controls the introduction of this type of legislation). Mindful of prior failures, the major proponents (including the AFL-CIO and the Johnson administration) were willing to allow compromise to accomplish their basic goal. By contrast to Medicare Part A, the proposal to cover physician services (Medicare Part B) had its inception as a last minute alternative devised by the House Republican minority on Ways and Means (most notably Congressman John Byrnes) and was supported by the American Medical Association (AMA) as a substitute for the administration's proposal. As a result, the details of

Part B, and most notably the methodology for physician payment, have not been carefully studied.

As noted before, the proposed Medicare reimbursement mechanism was based on the UCR methodology that had been used by a few private insurance programs. It is important to note that there were very sketchy data on what physicians' "customary" or "usual" charges were for most services since the UCR systems were new and data collection was minimal.

Another important factor was the involvement of the American Medical Association, which had played a major role in defeating national health insurance several times and was strongly opposed to the administration's proposal for mandatory hospital insurance. Indeed, some within the AMA advocated a boycott of the administration's program if it passed.[6] The AMA leadership, after some heated debates, decided to pursue a course strongly opposing Medicare, while working behind the scenes to ensure that if it did pass, it would be favorable to physicians. These efforts, the desire of the advocates to ensure passage of Part A, and the wish of Congressman Wilbur Mills to put his own mark on the legislation (which gave rise to the so-called "three layer cake" of Medicare Parts A and B and Medicaid) resulted in a series of compromises and decisions that contributed to many of the problems related to the cost of physician services in the Medicare program.

Although unable to defeat Medicare Part A, the AMA's positions prevailed on nearly every aspect of the Part B program. Its most strongly held position related to the right of physicians to determine their own charges. This resulted in the language of the Medicare legislation that stipulated that physician reimbursement under Medicare would be some variant of the UCR methodology. The legislation stated: "In determining the reasonable charge . . . there shall be taken into consideration the customary charges for similar services generally made by the physicians or other person furnishing such services as well as the prevailing charges in the locality for similar services."[5]

In addition to voluntary participation by the elderly in Part B (it is voluntary, although 98 percent of those eligible for Part A enroll in Part B), the AMA also won the right for physicians to balance bill and to determine assignment on a case-by-case basis. Thus, unlike hospitals, home care agencies, and nursing homes, physicians may decide on a case-by-case basis whether or not to accept Medicare reimbursement as full payment for the services rendered. Another compromise won by the AMA was a phrase in the law that prohibited the government from any action that could be construed as interference in the practice of medicine or in the physician-patient relationship. This phrase was interpreted by some at the time (and since) to mean that the role of the Medicare program itself was simply to collect revenues and pay bills.

Another facet was to allow radiologists, anesthesiologists, and pathologists to bill Medicare or to bill the patient directly. There were even fewer data on the usual fees of this group since most of them were paid on a salary or contract basis by hospitals. Finally, a compromise extracted by the private insurance companies and favored by the AMA allowed much of the decision making about the level of allowable fees and about what claims should be paid to be decentralized to regional carriers (Part B), which turned out in most cases to be Blue Cross–Blue Shield companies. The carriers were given rather wide latitude not only in establishing allowable charge levels, but also in creating specialty and geographic variations in payment structure. As a result, one state, Texas, has thirty-eight separate fee areas, while eighteen states have only one reimbursement area. Likewise, there are some states, such as Florida and North and South Dakota, where no specialty differentials are recognized, while in Pennsylvania fifty-eight different specialties are recognized. Given all the possible combinations and permutations, it is no wonder that seldom do physicians or patients know how much Medicare will pay for any given service.[1]

It should be noted that those in the administration who were charged with the responsibility of implementing Medicare realized the inherent inflationary nature of this reimbursement system. Within the limits set by the legislation and report language, and under the close scrutiny of Congressman Mills and the AMA, several provisions were put into the regulations that were issued that would form the basis of later controls on physician fees. The regulations issued to invoke the legislation required that physicians be reimbursed an "allowable charge," which was the lesser of what they billed, their usual charge for that service (confusingly termed by Medicare as "customary"), the prevailing charge (analogous to the customary charge of the UCR system), or what was determined to be reasonable. The prevailing screen of this CPR system was originally set (like the customary screen of UCR) to the ninetieth percentile of the charges submitted for the service by other physicians. The physicians' own customary fees and the regions' prevailing fees were reset each year, based on the prior year's submitted charges. Uwe Rheinhart has observed that this "granted health care providers a license to take from the collective insurance treasuries what they pleased."[7]

MEDICARE EXPENDITURES AND THE CPR SYSTEM

Given the payment mechanism adopted and the previously unmet needs of the elderly, it is not surprising that expenditures for Part B services accelerated rapidly in the first few years of Medicare. As noted above, the problems with the system were exacerbated by the fact that there were virtually no data on prevailing or customary fees. In most cases Medicare paid whatever the physician decided to charge. As early as 1970 there was clear evidence that Medicare allowances were far exceeding what private insurers had been paying under fee schedules.[8, 9] The upward trend was further accelerated by the fact that most other insurers, including Blue Shield, quickly switched to the CPR/UCR methodology.[10] In the first three years of the program the rate of increase in physician services exceeded 25 percent per year. Over the period 1967–1986 the annual compound rate of growth in Medicare expenditures for physician services was 16 percent in absolute terms and almost 9 percent in real (inflation-adjusted) terms. The rate of growth in payments has been uneven within the medical profession, which is reflected in changes in relative net physician income. The average annual increases between 1975 and 1986 ranged from over 20 percent per year in ophthalmology, anesthesiology, radiology, and cardiovascular disease to a low of 12 percent in family and general practice.[2, 11]

Studies have shown that the proportion attributable to price versus volume increases also varies by specialty.[2, 11] The overall increases in some specialties, such as family practice, general surgery, and anesthesiology, have been due primarily to medical price inflation, while in others, such as radiology, volume has been a much greater factor. Most of the specialties with the highest overall increases (thoracic surgery, cardiology, and ophthalmology) have shown increases in both volume and price. Since most payers have a payment structure similar to Medicare, the overall result has been that since 1970, while physician incomes in the aggregate have fallen by 4 percent (adjusted for inflation), those in family medicine have fallen by nearly 20 percent, and those for anesthesiologists, radiologists, and general surgeons have risen by 10 to 20 percent more than inflation.[12, 13] Note that this increase in net physician income for specialists (after malpractice and other practice expenses) has occurred in the face of a rapid increase in the number of physicians and most especially those in specialty areas.

THE EVOLUTION FROM PASSIVE PAYER TO PRUDENT PURCHASER

At the time of the enactment of Medicare, the major goal was to increase the access of the elderly to medical care services. As a result of this emphasis, the agency responsible for the administration of the program was initially viewed more as a passive collection and distribution center than as a purchaser of medical care. Partly as a result of the rapid increases in program expenditures and, in a few instances, in concerns about the quality of care, Congress initiated a series of actions that gradually transformed Medicare from passive payer to prudent purchaser.

As mentioned above, when the Medicare program was first established, the ninetieth percentile of prevailing fees was set as one limit of the Medicare allowable charge. In 1967–1970 this limit was reduced to the seventy-fifth percentile. In addition, in 1973 the yearly increase in prevailing fees was limited by the imposition of the "adjusted" prevailing fee. The adjustment was the Medicare Economic Index or MEI, an index related to practice expenses (40 percent) and general earnings increases of nonagricultural workers (60 percent). The seventy-fifth percentile of prevailing fees in effect in June 1973 is adjusted yearly by this index. The lesser of this adjusted prevailing fee or the seventy-fifth percentile of the actual prevailing fee is used as the limit. Nearly 85 percent of all actual charges submitted by physicians are reduced by the prevailing or adjusted prevailing fee, with the average reduction totaling 20 percent. Thus, most physicians (or patients, where claim assignment is not accepted) are currently being reimbursed by Medicare on the basis of the prevailing fee structure present in 1973 in a given region and/or specialty, adjusted for increases in earnings and office expenses.[3]

For new services, the Medicare allowable charge is based largely on the charges that have been submitted by the physicians to a given carrier prior to the time that the procedure is recognized as reimbursable by Medicare. Some decisions are made at the carrier level, although the Health Care Financing Administration (HCFA), acting on the recommendations of the Office of Health Technology Assessment, generally makes decisions on whether major new technologies should be reimbursed. After a prevailing charge is established, it is subsequently updated in the same manner as for older services. Obviously, physicians who develop and implement new procedures have a much greater opportunity to control the allowable charge level than do those who rely on established procedures. Note that there is no incentive for decreasing the level of charges if the procedure becomes less expensive to perform over time (in terms of time or materials). Thus, coronary bypass surgery, which initially required many hours and was done by only a very few surgeons, has not decreased in price despite the fact that some surgical teams now perform several each day.[3]

In 1984 Congress passed a number of provisions in the Deficit Reduction Act (DEFRA) that further modified physician reimbursement. The most notable action was a fee freeze, which eliminated the scheduled updates of the prevailing charges and subsequent recognition of customary charges until October 1985. (This freeze was extended until May 1986 for participating physicians and until January 1987 for other physicians.) In addition, the act established the participating physician program in which, in exchange for the agreement to accept assignment of payment for all Medicare patients, physicians would be reimbursed more promptly, could recognize charge increases when the freeze was lifted (although they could not collect any more than the Medicare allowable amount during the freeze), and would be listed as participating physicians in materials made available to Medicare recipients. In 1986 Congress took further steps to limit the increase in charges to Medicare patients by nonparticipating physicians (by the so-called maximum allowable actual charge or MAAC, which limited the amount by which nonparticipating physicians could increase their actual charges), established a statutory basis for reducing allowable charges based on "inherent reasonableness," and then actually reduced the allowable charges for a number of specific procedures (most notably cataract surgery). The concept of inherently reasonable was further extended in 1987 and 1988, with clarification of the conditions under which it could be applied and with further specific reductions in allowable (prevailing) charges. These latter actions are evidence of the growing recognition by Congress that Medicare is a major purchaser of physician services. Indeed, for some services like cataract surgery, pacemaker insertion, hip and knee replacement, and prostatectomy, Medicare accounts for over 75 percent of the market.[3]

Despite all the changes, there is little evidence to date that expenditures on physicians' services have been moderated. Even the imposition of the freeze did not seem to slow the rate of rise, and further it affected disproportionately those areas where price, rather than service volume and intensity, has been the driving force.[2] The adjusted prevailing fee, the Medicare Economic Index, the participating physician program, and the maximal allowable charge program have also had little apparent effect on expenditure levels, while adding further complexity to an already confusing system. Despite all the negatives of the CPR system, even the most ardent foe would have to admit that it has created almost universal access for Medicare beneficiaries, albeit at no small cost. Discrimination against the elderly in the provision of medical care services covered by Medicare is rare, and many feel that the extent of acute medical care of the elderly in the United States is unparalleled.

In recognition of the increasing complexity of physician reimbursement and the unabated rise in the costs of Part B of Medicare, in 1986 Congress mandated a Physician Payment Review Commission (PPRC) to provide advice to Congress concerning physician reimbursement under Medicare. Just six months after it was established, the commission was able to issue a preliminary report and has quickly assumed a major role in the continuing efforts to make Medicare a more prudent purchaser of physician services.[14, 15] The development of the PPRC, the creation of the Prospective Payment Advisory Commission (ProPAC), and the introduction of the prospective payment system for hospitals, along with the enhanced data analysis and review by the HCFA, are perhaps the final recognitions that the Medicare program is anything but a passive payer.

BEYOND CPR: REVOLUTION OR INCREMENTAL CHANGE

A number of initiatives outside the Medicare program have indirectly affected Medicare physician reimbursement. Beginning with the Nixon administration and greatly reinforced by the Reagan administration, there has been a growing emphasis on trying to enhance competition in medical care, primarily through the use of capitation.[16] Largely as a result of this emphasis, until 1984 HMOs participating in Medicare were paid for both hospital and physician services like any other entity on the basis of allowable costs or charges. This discouraged HMOs from making efforts to enroll Medicare patients since many of the closed-panel plans did not have an adequate system of tracking and billing physician charges. In 1984 Medicare law was changed to allow the establishment of Medicare risk contracts for HMOs and community health plans that permitted capitation payments to HMOs for services to Medicare patients. Obviously, the major advantage of capitation is the ability to prospectively budget and limit overall expenditures. However, because of limitations in the method developed to determine the level of the Medicare capitation payment, the inability of the HMO to pass any savings directly to the consumer (except in the form of increased benefits), the marked heterogeneity of the health risks of the Medicare population (which increases the possibility of favorable or unfavorable selection of patients by HMOs), and the tendency of patients with chronic illnesses to remain with their "own" physician, the use of HMOs by Medicare beneficiaries has lagged well behind their use by the public at large. In addition, the well-publicized problems of International Medical Centers (IMC) of Florida, an HMO with one of the largest enrollments of Medicare patients, have further dampened the enthusiasm of the elderly for physician services in capitated systems.

Moreover, since many of the newer HMOs enrolling Medicare patients are independent practice associations (IPAs), it is not clear whether payments to physicians have been changed by the introduction of capitation into Medicare. While most closed-panel group- or staff-model HMOs pay physicians a salary with some incentive income based on the service utilization or profitability of the HMO, some IPAs base physician payments on either a fee schedule or a reduced fee-for-service basis. Concerns raised by the AMA and elderly advocacy groups resulted in Congress' mandating a study of incentive payments to physicians in Medicare HMOs. In addition, the tendency of physicians in capitated arrangements to underprovide services may be of special concern in the substantial minority of older persons who have serious chronic illnesses and who are poorly equipped to "jump the hurdles" imposed by many capitated systems.

Some HMOs have experienced favorable selection (i.e., they have enrolled Medicare patients who are on average healthier than their age, sex, and Medicaid status cohort), and as a result the Medicare risk contract program may have cost Medicare more than an equivalent in the fee-for-service system.[17] Despite this finding tending to favor HMOs, the number of HMOs with Medicare risk contracts has grown much more slowly than anticipated. In an attempt to extend the concept of capitated reimbursement to chronic illness, the HCFA has funded an interesting experiment (called the social HMO or SHMO), which attempts to cover some long-term care services with a small premium added to the basic Medicare program.[18]

Another means of paying physicians for Medicare services that has been proposed is the bundling or grouping of services by diagnosis.[19, 20] It should be noted that the legislation that created the prospective payment system for hospitals (based on diagnosis-related groups or DRGs) mandated that the HCFA study the possibility of extending the DRG payment methodology to physician services. The essence of the system as applied to physicians would be to pay physicians (or, more likely, hospitals or physician groups) a prospectively set amount for all services rendered for a patient (during a hospitalization or an episode of illness, or for some fixed time) based on the diagnosis of the patient. A proposal by the Reagan administration would have reimbursed radiologists, anesthesiologists, and pathologists under Medicare by means of such diagnosis-related groups. The proposal was strongly opposed by the AMA and went nowhere in Congress. A major problem with the DRG methodology when applied to physician services— and especially to services for the frail, multiply impaired older person—is the lack of correlation between the intensity of physician services and the diagnosis of the patient. Nowhere is this more evident than in the care of patients in nursing homes where diagnosis alone explains very little of the need for physician services. In addition, it would create, as has DRG-based hospital reimbursement, a system of revenue winners and losers that would encourage physicians to care for those persons with less severe disease.

In addition to capitation, DRGs, and fee-for-service, there have been attempts by the HCFA to explore the possibility of competitive contracts for Medicare physician services, either with so-called preferred provider organizations (PPOs) or with other physician groups or hospitals. Such contracts could be limited to specific services (some private insurers, for example, have contracted for coronary bypass surgery with a specific group) or extended to all physician services. In essence, this is a variation of a negotiated fee schedule, but one that might vary considerably in different parts of the country. One of the main concerns is that there might be a lack of competition in many areas of the country. In addition, such a system would require close monitoring to see that all contract services were pro-vided in a timely and high-quality manner. Further, without some overall limit on expenditures for a given group (which would then be a form of capitation), this approach would not address the problem of volume. The experience of the government in the area of defense contracting does not augur well for this approach to Medicare reimbursement.

As noted in the first part of this chapter, the concept of a fee schedule is not new, having been the predominant mode of reimbursement for physi-cians under Blue Shield plans prior to the implementation of Medicare. Indeed, the use of the prevailing charge limit in Medicare has created de facto a charge-based Medicare fee schedule for most physicians. Fee sched-ules have usually been based on either historical charges or a negotiated amount.[21] The use of a fee schedule based on historical costs (or prevailing charge limits) would essentially enshrine existing inequities. The concept of a payment system based on the imputed cost of resources used by a physician in delivering is relatively new, having been espoused chiefly by William C. Hsiao and his coworkers at Harvard.[22] The major argument used by Hsiao in support of a resource-based relative-value scale (RBRVS) is an economic one. If one had a truly competitive system, and if charges exceeded resource costs, the profit generated would attract competitors. Conversely, if charges were less than resource costs, there would be a net loss and eventually a decrease in competitors. In essence, the RBRVS considers the relative work of physicians (including time and intensity) and the costs of practice (including costs for prior training, malpractice, and office personnel) in producing a given service within a given specialty. Using a series of cross-linkages (services provided by more than one specialty or judged by a physician panel as being equivalent), the system adjusts and relates relative values across different specialties. Except for redistributing income among physicians and perhaps reducing the incentives to do inappropriate or unnecessary procedures, the RBRVS would do nothing to control Medicare expenditures.

In order to create a fee schedule from an RBRVS, a base multiplier would be established which, when multiplied by a given relative value, would produce a fee. For example, if an appendectomy has a relative value of 3.4 and if the base multiplier is $100, the allowable fee for an appendectomy is $340. The Hsiao study does not address the question of how to establish the base amount, when and how the base amount should be updated, whether the base amount should be adjusted for geographic or specialty area, or whether the physician should be required to accept the Medicare fee as full payment (i.e., mandated assignment). All of these issues will affect the quality of care, out-of-pocket expenses for the elderly, equity for physicians, and access to services, as well as total expenditures by the Medicare program. It has also been noted by the PPRC[14] and others that a fee schedule would not address the element most responsible in recent years for the rapid rise in Medicare payments to physicians—namely, the volume and intensity of services—and especially in payments for new technology. Yet the establishment of a fee schedule, however derived, does give the administration and Congress the potential for more control over Medicare physician expenditures, especially through control of the updating of the base multiplier.

A variety of proposals to address overall expenditures have been advanced. The more interesting ones include prospective regional capitation, in which a geographically defined area of the country would receive a prospectively determined amount of money for physician services, and the use of expenditure targets, in which the base multiplier in the fee schedule would be adjusted upward or downward, depending on whether Medicare physician payments exceeded a prospectively determined target expenditure in the previous period. Thus, if the volume of physician services increased more than expected, the base multiplier could be raised less than inflation or even decreased.[23]

If the goals of the Medicare program are, indeed, to promote the delivery of quality health care services to beneficiaries, to make these services accessible to them, and to do so in a manner that is consistent with the cost-effective delivery of services within both the Medicare and the general U.S. health care system, what method of physician reimbursement best meets these goals? Or perhaps more to the point, given the goals of the Medicare system and the goals of all the interest groups (or, as some have termed them, self-interest groups) concerned with Medicare physician reimbursement, what is likely to happen?

There is a strong tradition of incrementalism in both American politics and health care. The most apparent reason for this incrementalism is the diversity of political forces acting on an issue at any one time. The considerable political power of taxpayers, as evidenced by recent actions and pronouncements by Congress and the administration, is focused on changing physician reimbursement primarily to the extent that it might reduce general revenue expenditures on Medicare Part B. This force will be balanced against the political activism of physicians who want to maintain their favorable economic status and of Medicare beneficiaries who want to maintain access and, at the same time, limit their out-of-pocket payments for deductibles, copayments, premiums, and, most especially, balance billing.

Much to the displeasure of physicians, measures such as expenditure targets or simply "savings" achieved by increases in the base multiplier for the fee schedule that are lower than inflation will be imposed to limit total Part B expenditures. Further measures will be introduced in the future to limit physician use of, and reimbursement for, new procedures. Hopefully, some of these constraints will be based to some degree on a better understanding of appropriateness and cost effectiveness.

In the end, and perhaps in the best tradition of pluralism, checks and balances, and other elements of our national character, it is likely that we will have a mixed system of fee-schedule-based fee-for-service reimbursement and capitated reimbursement. Perhaps this combination will produce a rational allocation of physician services with the potential disadvantage of each being limited and balanced by the competition between them.

NOTES

1. U.S. Congress, Office of Technology Assessment, *Payment for Physician Services: Strategies for Medicare*, OAT-H–294 (Washington, D.C.: U.S. Government Printing Office, 1986), pp. 37–77.

2. S. W. Letsch, K. R. Levit, and D. R. Waldo, "National Health Expenditures, 1987," *Health Care Financing Review* 10 (1988): 109–22.

3. D. Juba and M. B. Sulvetta, in J. F. Holahan and L. M. Etheredge, eds. *Medicare Physician Payment Reform—Issues and Options* (Washington, D.C.: Urban Institute Press, 1986), pp. 11–28.

4. J. A. Showstack et al., "Fee-for-Service Physician Payment: Analysis of Current Methods and Their Development," *Inquiry* 16 (1979): 230.

5. T. Marmor, *Politics of Medicine* (London: Routledge & Kegan-Paul, 1970).

6. F. D. Campion, *The AMA and U.S. Health Policy Since 1940* (Chicago: Chicago Review Press, 1984).

7. U. E. Reinhardt, "Resource Allocation in Health Care: The Allocation of Lifestyles to Providers," *Milbank Memorial Fund Quarterly* 65 (1987): 153–76.

8. K. M. Langwell and L. M. Nelson, "Physician Payment Systems: A Review of History, Alternatives and Evidence," *Medical Care Review* 43 (1986): 5–58.

9. F. A. Sloan and J. W. Hay, "Medicare Pricing Mechanisms for Physician Services: An Overview of Alternative Approaches," *Medical Care Review* 43 (1986): 59–100.

10. T. L. Delbanco, K. C. Meyers, and E. A. Segal, "Paying the Physician's Fee—Blue Shield and the Reasonable Charge," *New England Journal of Medicine* 301 (1979): 314–20.

11. L. Etheredge, in J. F. Holahan and L. M. Etheredge, eds., *Medicare Physician Payment Reform—Issues and Options* (Washington, D.C.: Urban Institute Press, 1986) pp. 125–51.

12. R. A. Reynolds and R. L. Ohsfeldt, eds., *Socioeconomic Characteristics of Medical Practice, 1984* (Chicago: American Medical Association, 1984).

13. M. L. Gonzalez, D. W. Emmons, and E. J. Slora, eds., *Socioeconomic Characteristics of Medical Practice, 1988* (Chicago: American Medical Association, 1988).

14. Physician Payment Review Commission, *Annual Report to Congress*—Medicare Physician Payment: An Agenda for Reform (Washington, D.C.: U.S. Government Printing Office, 1987).

15. Physician Payment Review Commission, *Annual Report to Congress* (Washington, D.C.: U.S. Government Printing Office, 1988).

16. U.S. Congress, Office of Technology Assessment, *Payment for Physician Services: Strategies for Medicare*, pp. 177–208.

17. H. S. Luft, "Compensating for Biased Selection in Health Insurance," *Milbank Memorial Fund Quarterly* 64 (1986): 566–91.

18. W. Leutz et al., "Targeting Expanded Care to the Aged: Early SHMO Experience," *Gerontologist* 28 (1988): 4–17.

19. U.S. Congress, Office of Technology Assessment, *Payment for Physician Services—Strategies for Medicare*, pp. 153–75.

20. S. F. Jencks and A. Dobson, "Strategies for Reforming Medicare's Physician Payments," *New England Journal of Medicine* 312 (1985): 1492–99.

21. U.S. Congress, Office of Technology Assessment, *Payment for Physician Services—Strategies for Medicare*, pp. 119–52.

22. W. C. Hsiao et al., "Estimating Physicians' Work for a Resource-Based Relative-Value Scale," *New England Journal of Medicine* 319 (1988): 835–41.

23. Physician Payment Review Commission, *Annual Report to Congress* (Washington, D.C.: U.S. Government Printing Office, 1989).

Conclusion: The Fruits of Reform—A New Payment Scheme

John F. Hoadley

In 1989 Congress made fundamental changes in the way Medicare will pay physicians. Over a period of five years, starting in 1992, the Medicare program will implement a fee schedule based on a resource-based relative-value scale (RBRVS) that will have major implications for how physicians do business. There will be winners and losers among the various medical specialties, and, for the first time, there will be limits on the actual charges paid by beneficiaries.

To students and observers of the legislative process, the most remarkable aspect of the passage of these changes is the relative speed with which they finally occurred. In 1983 Congress had also defied conventional wisdom in passing a comprehensive reform in the way Medicare pays hospitals. Together these two pieces of legislation constitute a substantial restructuring of Medicare—accomplished with surprisingly little fanfare.

For years the conventional wisdom in Washington and among students of the legislative process has been that Congress cannot easily confront the powerful medical establishment. The original creation of the Medicare and Medicaid programs was delayed for years by the lobbying of organized medicine. As recently as 1984 the American Medical Association (AMA) and its allies blocked limits on what physicians could charge their patients over and above Medicare-approved amounts (balance billing). The House of Representatives was sufficiently intimidated by organized medicine that its decision was taken by a voice vote, allowing members to avoid going on the record on the issue.

During the 1980s, however, politics changed in a variety of ways beyond the Republican stronghold in the White House. The most significant of these has been the dominance of the federal budget, both in the way that large deficits have limited the scope of policy making and in the way that the budget process has come to be the main locus for considering new policies and changes in existing programs.

THE CHANGING NATURE OF THE POLICY-MAKING PROCESS IN THE 1980s

For many policy issues, getting on the agenda is the easy part; actual policy making is far more difficult. The political landscape is littered with proposals like national health insurance and the Nixon guaranteed-income plan that never became law. The process, once described as the "obstacle course on Capitol Hill" (Bendiner, 1965), has blocked many proposals that enjoyed fairly widespread support.

The legislative process, according to conventional wisdom, works slowly and deliberately—especially when it comes to policies of any significance. One recent example of the deliberate nature of the process is the Tax Reform Act of 1986, which was signed into law more than a year after its introduction and several years after Senator Bill Bradley (D–N.J.) and Representative Richard Gephardt (D–Mo.) first floated the idea. Its passage came after an agonizingly long series of hearings on both sides of the Hill, after several pronouncements of its death, and after resuscitations performed by such key actors as Representative Dan Rostenkowski (D–Ill.) and Senator Bob Packwood (R–Ore.). Such legislative sagas have been repeated many times, including during the effort to pass the original Medicare legislation in 1965.

The textbook image of the legislative process also incorporates the passage of a limited number of bills that are less comprehensive than those of the scope of tax reform. Legislation would wend its slow way through the legislative process; in the health arena one could expect a handful of major bills to be enacted in most years.

But the pattern that persisted through the 1960s and 1970s hardly fits the legislative scene of the 1980s and 1990s. In recent times, most successful legislation—particularly in the health field—depends on a "fast-track" vehicle. I have discussed the use of the legislative fast track as a means to enact major legislation without benefit of lengthy or extended deliberation. In 1983 Congress enacted the reform of Medicare's method of paying hospitals by attaching it to a social security reform measure that was needed to solve a crisis in the social security trust funds (Fuchs and Hoadley, 1984). In 1985 Congress passed the Gramm-Rudman-Hollings deficit reduction package as an amendment to the "must pass" bill to increase the public debt limit (Hoadley, 1986). In both of these cases, streamlined procedures and the commitment of key congressional actors made possible the speedy passage of legislation that might otherwise have faced extended delay and possible defeat.

The use of fast-track legislative vehicles for the passage of major policy initiatives remains more the exception than the rule, although in a conservative antigovernment administration, there are few opportunities to test the rule. What is perhaps more remarkable is that fast-track vehicles have become nearly the only legislative vehicles in the health policy arena. A few relatively noncontroversial bills (such as that to increase funds for AIDS research) and a limited set of relatively routine reauthorizations of existing programs (such as that to support community health centers) are permitted traditional routes through the legislative process.

But the watchword for most proposals is "wait for reconciliation." Budget reconciliation legislation has become the vehicle for most new proposals in health policy. Since 1980, reconciliation bills have become an annual exercise in deficit reduction. Indeed, reconciliation is the principal means by which Congress can achieve changes in those entitlement programs that are not included in the traditional appropriations process. Whereas discretionary programs (such as health research or the National Health Service Corps) can be funded at higher or lower levels through annual appropriations bills, any change in an entitlement program (such as Medicare) requires an amendment to the law that created that entitlement. Reconciliation is the legislative vehicle for making such changes in law (Ellwood, 1985).

In terms of the legislative process, reconciliation instructions are included in the annual budget resolution passed by Congress in the spring of each year. These instructions indicate to the various congressional committees the dollar amounts of budget savings they are required to produce in programs under their jurisdiction. Each committee proceeds to mark up its reconciliation provisions during the summer and report back to the Budget Committee. The Budget Committee then assembles these items into an omnibus reconciliation bill which (in theory) is debated and passed by the October 1 start of the new fiscal year. The result of this process in the past several years is a series of bills best known by such acronyms as OBRA, DEFRA, and COBRA.

In the early 1980s, reconciliation bills were generally restricted to provisions that produced budget savings, but legislators soon realized that these bills were unlikely targets of presidential vetoes and thus ripe opportunities for their pet projects. As a result, the more recent bills have been loaded with a wide variety of legislative provisions and have provided the route to passage for substantial reforms in the Medicare and Medicaid programs. In fact, these legislative packages have come to dominate the final stages of most annual sessions of Congress, often climaxing in showdowns between the president and Congress.

In spite of the popularity of these extraneous provisions, committee chairmen have attempted to limit them by enforcing budget neutrality—meaning that any amendment to the package must retain equal budget savings. An additional impediment was added in 1986 when the Senate forbade, among others, all provisions that had *no* budget impact (known as the Byrd rule). Further procedural changes were added under Gramm-Rudman-Hollings. The result is an arsenal of tools available to chairmen or other committee members who are opposed to adding new items to a package.

The use of budget reconciliation as the main way to pass health legislation has significant implications for policy making and for the legislative process. It has quickened the pace of deliberations, moved much of these deliberations behind closed doors, imposed tight budget constraints on the set of alternatives, curbed outside influence, and altered relationships between the executive and legislative branches. More generally, it has fundamentally transformed the policy making process in the health arena.

THE CASE OF PROSPECTIVE PAYMENT FOR HOSPITALS

The enactment of a hospital prospective payment system (PPS) in 1983 must be regarded as a major restructuring of the Medicare system.[1] Under the former system a hospital was reimbursed for whatever costs were incurred in the treatment of a patient, with only a few limitations. This retrospective system had the unfortunate effect of creating incentives for hospitals to administer too many tests, to keep patients longer than necessary, and to find ways to increase revenues, often in the name of more thorough care. The new system was designed to reverse these financial incentives by establishing a set level of reimbursement for a given diagnosis or, more specifically, for a diagnosis-related group (DRG). If the hospital provides treatment at a lower cost, it can keep the difference; if the bill for a particular patient is higher than the set DRG payment, the hospital must bear the additional cost.

This major reform, with enormous consequences for American hospitals, was enacted as an amendment to the Social Security Amendments of 1983 (Public Law 98–21), the law that rescued social security from bankruptcy. The social security package was a classic piece of "must pass" legislation and was described by one participant as "one of the greatest legislative engines we'll ever see" (Iglehart, 1983, p. 1430). While there was considerable public debate over the social security rescue plan, there was very little attention to or debate over the adoption of the prospective payment system. Swift passage was also aided by the fact that the DRG system became all things to all people, being described in floor debate by one member of Congress as an important first step toward competition in health care and by another as "good" regulation.

The rapid and relatively noncontroversial enactment of such a substantial reform of a major program like Medicare appeared to deny the conventional wisdom about congressional policy making. Given the traditional status and power of the medical community in the political arena, it is remarkable that such a reform would occur without intense public scrutiny or presidential pressure.

THE CONTEXT OF PHYSICIAN PAYMENT REFORM

In 1988 physicians received nearly $25 billion from the federal Medicare program; Medicare payments represent close to one-fourth of the income physicians earn each year. During the decade of the 1980s Medicare's total spending on physician services rose by 15 to 18 percent per year (Alston, 1989; Rovner, 1989a).

This steady rate of increase has been a significant concern to federal policymakers for several years. Observers and participants were heard to say regularly that "this is the year of the physician." But comprehensive reform did not see action throughout most of the decade. A number of marginal changes were made, but they left the question of comprehensive reform unanswered.

When Medicare was created in 1965, Congress approved a fee system that was viewed by most observers as favorable to physicians. The customary, prevailing, and reasonable (CPR) payment system, similar to that used by private insurers, paid a physician the lowest of the actual charge, his or her customary charge for the same service, or the prevailing charge for that service among other physicians in a specific area. While this system placed some limits on fees, doctors were able to control the increase of fees because their fees drove changes in the customary and prevailing rates. In addition, physicians were permitted to bill patients for any charges that exceeded the Medicare-approved amount.

The only significant change in the system of paying physicians in the first fifteen years under Medicare came in 1972 when Congress placed an inflation cap on allowed physician charges. After the CPR methodology was applied to ascertain an allowed charge, this amount was capped by a rate of increase based on the Medicare Economic Index (MEI). While the effect of this cap was not dramatic, it did place some limit on the rate of growth.

From the mid-1970s through the mid-1980s, Congress was unsuccessful in efforts to restructure Medicare as a whole or to make significant changes in the way physicians were paid. The next legislative action aimed at limiting the growth of physician expenditures was the freeze on fees, imposed initially from July 1, 1984, to October 1, 1985. The freeze was enacted as part of the Deficit Reduction Act of 1984 (DEFRA, Public Law 98–369), which also established a system of participating physicians, defined as those who agreed to accept the Medicare-approved fee as payment in full for all patients.

Before the freeze ended, Congress—in the Consolidated Omnibus Budget Reconciliation Act (COBRA, Public Law 99–272)—extended it until May 1, 1986, for participating physicians and until January 1, 1987, for nonparticipating physicians. After years of defeat by allies of the powerful medical establishment, the fee freeze marked the first significant victory for advocates of physician payment reform. In fact, Congress went a step farther in allowing fees to rise somewhat faster for participating physicians than for nonparticipating doctors.

One additional provision was included in COBRA: creation of the Physician Payment Review Commission (PPRC). This new legislative-branch agency was charged with making recommendations to Congress on potential reforms in the way physicians are paid under Medicare. Congress also requested that the Department of Health and Human Services (DHHS) report on the feasibility of enacting a new payment mechanism employing a relative-value scale that would rank the value of doctors' services by the amount of time, training, and overhead required to provide them.

The net effect of these changes was to put a process in motion that would eventually lead to a more fundamental reform of the system. The fee freeze established the fact that Congress was prepared to take serious action to control rising expenditures for physicians services. In addition, the participating physician program represented the first time that Congress had limited in any way balance billing—what physicians could collect from their patients. Finally, Congress had requested reports from two agencies on more comprehensive reforms.

The next two budget cycles marked a continuation of the incremental approach to physician payment reform. In the Omnibus Budget Reconciliation Act of 1986 (OBRA–86, Public Law 99–509), Congress created a complicated system of maximum allowable actual charges (MAACs). This system was designed to place some limits on what nonparticipating physicians could charge their patients, while allowing other physicians to bring their fees more in line with those of their colleagues. In addition, DHHS was authorized to reduce the Medicare-approved charge for certain procedures (such as cataract surgery) that it deemed to be overpriced.

In 1987 Congress passed as part of OBRA–87 (Public Law 100–203) several additional provisions that would affect physician payment. These included larger fee increases for primary care services than for other services and a larger differential between participating and nonparticipating physicians. Based on recommendations from the PPRC—which by now was making annual recommendations to Congress—fees were reduced for twelve surgical procedures considered to be overpriced.

By the end of 1987 two key series of events were under way that would eventually lead to physician payment reform. First, Congress had created an increasingly complicated set of controls to attempt to limit rising expenditures. Physicians were dealing with different fees for participating and nonparticipating physicians, MAACs, and higher fees for some procedures and reduced fees for others. The result, in the eyes of doctors, was a bewildering set of regulations and reduced autonomy in their practice of medicine. At the same time, however, expenditures were continuing to grow at a high rate. Spending had dipped slightly during the fee freeze, but research revealed that physicians had increased their volume of services to compensate for the frozen price of an individual service. Most policymakers were coming to the conclusion that incremental change was inadequate to reverse the spending trend.

The second critical series of events included the charges to the PPRC and DHHS to report back with recommendations for reform of the system. The resource-based relative-value scale (RBRVS) was the methodology that had attracted the greatest attention from policymakers (although a DRG system for physicians was also popular). Developed by William C. Hsiao and his colleagues at Harvard University, this yardstick measured the resources—including work, training, and overhead costs—that go into different services. The AMA was among the supporters of the research on the RBRVS, even though the new approach was not pleasing to all groups of physicians.

Just as with the events leading up to enactment of hospital payment reforms under Medicare, dissatisfaction on all sides with incremental changes and congressional requests for outside recommendations provided the basis for a consensus on reform. While the RBRVS was by no means a panacea, it provided a starting point for many different interests.

In research on the RBRVS, Hsiao and his colleagues concluded that certain procedures—especially those for surgery and diagnostic tests—were paid at too high a rate, while other procedures—such as primary care—were undervalued. These findings had the potential to divide the medical community into winners and losers, ensuring the opposition of at least some segments of organized medicine.

But there was also some skepticism on Capitol Hill, as reflected in the comments of Representative Fortney H. (Pete) Stark (D–Calif.), chairman of the Ways and Means Health Subcommittee. Turning the RBRVS into a fee schedule "is taking the existing pie and cutting it up into different size slices. The question is [how] you get the size of the whole pie down" (Rovner, 1989, p. 391). The experience under the fee freeze, when doctors compensated for lower fees by performing more procedures, was very much in the minds of policymakers.

ENACTING A MAJOR REFORM

In 1989 the pieces appeared to be in place to enact a reform of the way Medicare pays physicians.[2] In March the PPRC made its recommendations for a fee schedule based on an RBRVS, with adjustments for differences in practice costs by geographic region (Physician Payment Review Commission, 1989). The commission also included recommendations for expenditure targets (ETs) and for limits on balance billing.

ETs represented an attempt to control growth in the volume of services rendered by physicians. Under this plan a national target would be set each year for total Medicare spending on physician services, reflecting increases in practice costs, increases in the number of Medicare enrollees, and the appropriate rate of increase in the volume of services per enrollee. If actual costs exceeded the target, the inflation increase in fees for the next year would be reduced to make up the difference. Under the proposed balance-billing limits, physicians would eventually be precluded from charging more than 115 percent of the approved fee and could not collect any more than that amount from their patients.

A congressional hearing quickly revealed the range of opinions on the reform proposals. At an April 17 hearing of the Subcommittee on Health of the House Committee on Ways and Means, representatives of the American Academy of Family Physicians (AAFP), the American College of Physicians (ACP), and the American Society of Internal Medicine (ASIM) all expressed support for the basic RBRVS plan. They differed, however, on the ET plan. Representatives of both ACP and ASIM criticized ETs on the grounds that they would ultimately lead to long lines and denial of care. The AAFP witness, on the other hand, was not so concerned, saying that ETs would do little more than make explicit a process that was already under way with inflation updates under the existing fee schedule.

The AMA made the ET proposal its key lobbying target, calling it "implicit rationing" and "an unwarranted intrusion into the physician-patient relationship" (McIlrath, 1989, p. 47). In spite of the pressure, the Ways and Means Subcommittee on June 14 approved by an 11–3 vote a package that followed substantially the PPRC recommendations.

The Bush administration did not take long to respond. Two days after the subcommittee action, Louis Sullivan, Secretary of Health and Human Services, announced his support for the approach at a hearing of the Subcommittee on Medicare and Long-Term Care of the Senate Committee on Finance. But at its annual meeting in late June, the AMA launched an all-out effort to defeat the ET proposal. While reiterating its support for a fee schedule based on the RBRVS, it urged physicians to lobby Congress for the removal of ETs from the plan. With all the attention to ETs, organized medicine was saying little about the third component of the legislative proposal: limits on balance billing.

Meanwhile, under strong lobbying pressure, the legislative process continued to move along. Three congressional committees have jurisdiction over physician payment provisions under Medicare Part B: the Senate Committee on Finance, the House Committee on Energy and Commerce, and the House Committee on Ways and Means. The dual jurisdiction in the House provided a second chance for interest groups not happy with the decision of the first committee, and it created additional complications once a measure reached a conference committee at the end of the process.

When the full Ways and Means Committee took action, one key change was to provide separate expenditure targets for surgery and for all other services. The American College of Surgeons (ACS) had never allied itself with the AMA's fight against ETs, stating its support for the approach on the condition that surgery would get a separate target. Such a change would ensure that surgeons would not lose revenue relative to their colleagues.

With that one change, the Ways and Means package was approved on June 28. The only recorded vote came on a motion to strike the ET provision; it lost by 11 to 25. Bill Gradison (R-Ohio), ranking Republican on the health subcommittee, commented after the vote: "I am proud of the Ways and Means Committee for not being intimidated by the AMA's obvious attempt to scare the frail elderly" (Rovner, 1989b, p. 1627).

The next day, action came from the other House committee of jurisdiction. The Energy and Commerce Subcommittee on Health and the Environment approved its own plan to overhaul physician payments. The fee schedule and balance-billing limits resembled those in the Ways and Means bill, but the subcommittee did not include expenditure targets in the package. Said Subcommittee Chairman Henry A. Waxman (D-Calif.), ETs "would simply ratchet down on everybody, and that strikes me as unfair." He went on to say that he held this view "in spite of [the AMA's] ad campaign, not because of it" (Rovner, 1989b, p. 1627). The full committee on Energy and Commerce ratified the subcommittee plan on July 13.

At this point, action shifted to the Senate side. The House actions assured that ETs would have to be considered by the conference committee, but the outcome was unclear. The RBRVS fee schedule, however, appeared to be a sure thing. When Congress returned from its August recess, the key health policy issue was not physician payment reform, but repeal of the Medicare Catastrophic Coverage Act. The controversy over whether to repeal this law in full or to create a scaled-down benefit was much on the minds of Medicare beneficiaries, so members of Congress returned from their home districts convinced that the issue had to be resolved.

Meanwhile, the budget process was looming. With a new fiscal year beginning on October 1, Congress was under pressure to come up with its package of budget cuts to avoid automatic spending cuts under the Gramm-Rudman-Hollings deficit reduction procedures. Thus, to a great extent physician payment reform was once again on the back burner: Many observers predicted that another budget cycle would come and go without action.

Nevertheless, the process did not come to a halt. With several physician groups suggesting that a program of practice guidelines be substituted for the expenditure targets, the Senate Finance Committee began its consideration of physician payment reform. Senators John D. Rockefeller IV (D-W.Va.) and Dave Durenberger (R-Minn.), the two ranking members of the committee's Medicare subcommittee, came forth with what they hoped could be a compromise plan. Instead of ETs, they would set Medicare volume performance standards (MVPSs) that did not include automatic fee adjustments if total expenditures exceeded the standards.

After the full Finance Committee approved the Rockefeller-Durenberger plan on October 2, the *American Medical News* (McIlrath, 1989b) headlined its story, "Senators Reject ETs." Many observers believed it likely that the MVPS plan would form the basis of a final compromise, but it was not altogether clear what the committee had created in this new plan. The key provision appeared to be the elimination of the automatic fee adjustments called for by the ET proposal, with the MVPSs serving as an advisory guideline rather than a target set in law.

With the AMA declaring victory, the next question was whether the reforms would become law after all. In the maneuvering over the shape of the final budget agreement, the catastrophic insurance program, capital gains, and a wide variety of other issues threatened to tie Congress in knots. Prior to going to conference, the Senate chose to strip its reconciliation bill of all so-called extraneous provisions—including its recently passed physician payment reform package, which was estimated to be budget-neutral.

Therefore, when the House-Senate conference was formed, they were able to look at only two versions of physician payment: those passed by Ways and Means and by Energy and Commerce. Furthermore, Senate conferees were urging their House colleagues to agree to a stripped-down final package and leave the extraneous items for the next year. Pete V. Domenici (R-N.M.), ranking Republican on the Senate Budget Committee, said, "My proposal . . . was, go all the way and strip the bill of everything and set the precedent that this reconciliation bill in the Senate . . . is no longer going to be an omnibus bill [for] everything under the sun" (Calmes and Elving, 1989, p. 2691).

Eventually negotiations proceeded as if the Senate provisions were in the conference. In addition to the official conference document that described current law and both the House and the Senate versions as passed in each chamber, an unofficial conference document added the provisions as passed by the various Senate committees. Conferees thus had easy access to these items even though they were officially not part of the deliberations. Nevertheless, except to a handful of interested members of Congress, physician payment reform was hardly high on the political agenda at this point.

After over a month of stalemate over the high-profile issues, the budget agreement finally began to take shape, and physician payment reform was not part of it. On November 17, the committee leadership declared it dead, concluding that no agreement was possible in the few remaining days before Congress would adjourn for the year. This conclusion did not come as a great surprise to congressional observers. Even with the help of the legislative fast track, the issues involved in physician payment reform did not lend themselves to easy compromise.

But Senator Rockefeller (among others) decided he wanted a provision in the final bill.

"I was told it was dead and lay off it," [Rockefeller] said in an interview Nov. 22. "But I wasn't going to stand for it. It was ridiculous." So the next day—Saturday, Nov. 18—Rockefeller called together in Durenberger's conference room ("because he had a big enough table") the principal members and staff from both chambers and both parties, along with the Bush administration's chief expert on the issue, deputy domestic policy adviser William Roper. Working all day and into the night, the group ultimately hammered out an agreement that fell apart and came together at least three more times before the conference report on the bill finally reached the House and Senate floors in the early hours of Nov. 22. (Rovner, 1989c, p. 3240)

This closed-door, small-group effort was not atypical of the process by which the final shape of legislation is produced in Congress these days. The fact that a compromise had been reached in the waning hours of the session was generally known as the final votes occurred, but the exact shape of that agreement was probably understood by only a very few policymakers and the lobbyists whose job it was to know what was happening.

THE COMPONENTS OF PHYSICIAN PAYMENT REFORM

As incorporated in the Omnibus Budget Reconciliation Act of 1989 (OBRA–89), approved by Congress on November 22, 1989, and signed into law by the president (Public Law 102–239), physician payment reform includes the following major sections:

- Beginning in 1992 payment for physician services will be based on the lesser of the actual charge or the amount determined by the fee schedule.
- Payment under the fee schedule will equal the product of the relative value of the service, the conversion factor, and the geographic adjustment factor. Nonparticipating physicians will be paid at 95 percent of the fee-schedule amount.
- In determining relative values of physician services, DHHS will take into consideration the work component (physician time and intensity), the practice expense component (resources used—office rent, wages), and the malpractice component for each service that is provided.
- The conversion factor for each year will be the conversion factor for the previous year adjusted by the update for the year involved. The first year's (1992) conversion factor is calculated to yield budget neutrality.
- Each year, the secretary of DHHS will submit a recommended update factor. Congress will determine the final update factor.
- The geographic adjustment factor is calculated to reflect geographic variations in the costs of practice, malpractice, and physician work.
- Annual updates in the conversion factor for the fee schedule should be made based on the MVPS. The secretary and the PPRC will make recommendations for the

MVPS based on the changes in the number of beneficiaries, inflation, changes in volume and technology, and other factors.

- The default update is the predicted inflation increase, plus or minus the difference between actual performance and the year's performance standard, but the update could not be reduced by more than 3 percentage points (2 or 2.5 points in the transition years).
- Beginning in 1991 the secretary must recommend a separate MVPS for surgery.
- Nonparticipating physicians may not bill Medicare patients in excess of certain balance-billing limits. After 1992 the limiting charge will be 115 percent of the recognized payment amount under Part B.
- Implementation of the new fee schedule will begin in 1992, with certain transition provisions (easing the changes for those charges more than 15 percent different from the new fee schedule) applying for the first four years. After 1995 all payments will be made on the basis of the national fee schedule.[3]

REACTIONS AND IMPLEMENTATION

As the dust from the final days of the congressional session began to clear, Congress watchers had a chance to sort out what had happened. Interested observers believe that Congress outlined a fairly clear policy, although many of the details remain to be worked out later. The best-worked-out segment of the new policy is the fee schedule that resulted from many months of research at the PPRC and elsewhere. The other components of the new law, according to close observers, are less well spelled out. In the case of volume performance standards, the details changed several times during congressional consideration, and analysts in the HFCA and the PPRC will be responsible for working out the details.

Congress has also left itself with a substantial role in future years, and no one should believe that this action represents the last word from Capitol Hill. Just as each annual decision on the amount of the PPS update factor for hospital payments becomes a new political decision with consequences for both the federal budget and the operating margins of hospitals, so, too, will the update in the new fee schedule become an annual political issue.

The various groups within organized medicine are already sounding off on the merits and demerits of the final package. The American College of Physicians, in its January 1990 magazine, congratulated itself on helping to shape a positive reform (Ball, 1990). The AMA was clearly pleased to have defeated expenditure targets, but according to Representative Gradison, the differences between ETs and MVPSs are mostly semantic: "They read differently, but they're almost the same in terms of their impact" (Rovner, 1989c, p. 3241). One observer also noted that the AMA membership may eventually accuse its leadership of being asleep on balance-billing limits— that in the end this provision, although not debated at length, may prove to be a very important one.

KEY CONCLUSIONS

The result of congressional decision making was a substantial overhaul of the system by which Medicare pays physicians. And while skeptics frequently doubted that any reform would be accomplished, the changes did become law. As with reform of Medicare hospital payments just a few years earlier, Congress enacted a major reform with relative ease. Several conclusions can be drawn from this set of events.

1. Earlier legislative actions helped speed the momentum of reform. As in the case of hospital payment restructuring, Congress took several initial steps to contain rising costs. The enactment of a freeze on fees, reduced fees for overpriced procedures, and MAACs were all aimed at reducing Medicare Part B expenditures. But they also had the effect of creating what physicians and some policymakers regarded as a complex and burdensome set of regulations. When they failed to have any significant effect on reducing expenditures, a consensus began to develop that the time for reform had arrived.

2. A second factor at work in reforming both hospital and physician payments was the availability of an approach to reform, with research under way on that approach. In 1983 the state of New Jersey had already experimented with a system of DRGs for paying hospitals. In 1989, research on the RBRVS gave policymakers a methodology that could be used to create a new fee schedule for physicians. As consensus developed on the need for reform, most parties looked to the RBRVS as the favored approach. It quickly was assumed that if reform was to succeed, the RBRVS would be at the center of that reform. The existence of an outside body making recommendations—DHHS in one case and the PPRC in the other—also helped Congress in its decision making. The PPRC's recommendations on physician payment reform helped to give a shape to the emerging consensus.

3. The splitting of the powerful physician lobby was a key factor in preventing unified opposition to any of the more controversial portions of the reform package. The RBRVS approach itself created both winners and losers among the physician community. The winners, such as internists and family physicians, quickly surfaced as enthusiastic supporters of reform, while surgeons and others who emerged as losers under the system were skeptical or downright opposed. In the case of expenditure targets, the surgeons saw a way to improve their position and ended up supporting a position that other physician groups vehemently resisted. These divisions gave members of Congress plenty of political cover to vote for reform (Alston, 1989).

4. The presence in the reform package of three major components—a fee schedule, expenditure targets (or the MVPS substitute), and balance-billing limits—probably strengthened the package as a whole. The PPRC and other

reform advocates saw each component of the package as vital to creating a successful system. But the result was also a package with political staying power. The surgeons, who were most vehemently opposed to the fee schedule, found protection in the creation of a separate expenditure target, and the AMA's focus on expenditure targets meant that it gave relatively little attention to balance-billing limits, normally a major lobbying target for organized medicine.

5. The presence of a fast-track legislative vehicle was an essential component in the ultimate success of reform. As with so many other legislative initiatives in the 1980s, the traditional, civics-book legislative process was closed off. The budget reconciliation process provided an alternative legislative vehicle for physician payment reform. Although the process nearly collapsed at more than one point, it ultimately provided both momentum and protection to a proposal that could easily have been blocked by powerful opposition.

6. The budget process itself tends to restrict debate on individual legislative provisions. Floor procedures, especially on the House side, generally do not permit votes on individual items. Committee decisions are ratified when the full chamber accepts the budget package as a whole, and conference agreements are usually accepted or rejected on a single up-or-down vote. Thus, senior committee members and their staffs have nearly total responsibility for the shape of a reform package. Their support in the case of physician payment reform made success much easier. By limiting the scope of debate to those members of Congress on the three key committees, opponents lost access to many potential allies.

7. The distraction of other competing issues also helped to limit the scope of debate over physician payment reform. Decisions regarding capital gains taxes, the degree of deficit reduction, and the repeal of the Medicare catastrophic insurance program all were dominating the headlines. Many members of Congress were probably scarcely aware of any legislative action on physician payment reform, thus further easing the path to passage.

8. Finally, political leadership contributed to the success of reform. The package had strong advocates on each of the key committees, individuals who were willing to make sure that physician payment reform was part of the 1989 budget reconciliation package. And during the final hours of the legislative session, Senator Rockefeller was among those who were willing to make reform a priority—to work late into the night—and see that it survived in the final package.

While the shape of physician payment reform legislation was the product of thoughtful research and negotiation among many interested parties, it was politics—and the unique shape of the legislative process of the 1980s— that eased its way to passage. Without some of the protecting factors that accompanied this legislation, 1990 or 1991—not 1989—might have been the year when Medicare physician payment reform finally was enacted by Congress.

NOTES

1. A more detailed discussion of the enactment of a Medicare prospective payment system for hospitals can be found in Fuchs and Hoadley (1984, 1987). See also Nexon (1987) for an additional view of these events.

2. Two sources for regular, detailed reports on the progress of this legislation through Congress are *Congressional Quarterly Weekly Report* and *American Medical News*, the latter published by the American Medical Association.

3. See *Congressional Quarterly Weekly Report* (1989) and Firshein (1989) for more detailed summaries.

REFERENCES

Alston, Chuck (1989). "Belt-Tightening in Medicare Pits Doctor vs. Doctor." *Congressional Quarterly Weekly Report* 47 (October 7, 1989): 2605–9.

Ball, John (1990). "Headquarters Report: The College and RBRVS—For the Record." *American College of Physicians Observer* 10 (January 1990): 2–3.

Bendiner, Robert (1965). *Obstacle Course on Capitol Hill*. New York: McGraw-Hill.

Calmes, Jackie, and Ronald D. Elving (1989). "Bipartisan Deal Set in Senate to Strip Down Deficit Bill." *Congressional Quarterly Weekly Report* 47 (October 14, 1989): 2691–95.

Congressional Quarterly Weekly Report (1989). "Deficit-Reduction Bill Offers Billion in Cuts." *Congressional Quarterly Weekly Report* 47 (December 16, 1989): 3442–53.

Ellwood, John W. (1985). "The Great Exception: The Congressional Budget Process in an Age of Decentralization." In Lawrence C. Dodd and Bruce I. Oppenheimer, eds., *Congress Reconsidered*, 3d ed. Washington: CQ Press, pp. 161–88.

Firshein, Janet, ed. (1989). "Legislative Summary: Health Related Provisions of H.R. 3299, Omnibus Budget Reconciliation Act of 1989." *Health Legislation and Regulation* 15: 49 (December 20, 1989): 3–12.

Fuchs, Beth C., and John F. Hoadley (1984). "The Remaking of Medicare: Congressional Policymaking on the Fast Track." Paper presented at the annual meeting of the Southern Political Science Association, Savannah, Georgia, November 3, 1984.

Fuchs, Beth C., and John F. Hoadley (1987). "Reflections from Inside the Beltway: How Congress and the President Grapple with Health Policy." *PS* 20 (Spring 1987): 212–20.

Hoadley, John F. (1986). "Easy Riders: Gramm-Rudman-Hollings and the Legislative Fast Track." *PS* 19 (Winter 1986): 30–36.

Iglehart, John K. (1983). "Medicare Begins Prospective Payment of Hospitals." *New England Journal of Medicine* 308 (June 9, 1983): 1428–32.

McIlrath, Sharon (1989a). "House Subcommittee Endorses Expenditure Targets for MD Pay." *American Medical News* 32 (June 23–30, 1989): 1, 44–47.

McIlrath, Sharon (1989b). "Senators Reject ETs." *American Medical News* 32 (October 13, 1989): 1, 41–43.

Nexon, David (1987). "The Politics of Congressional Health Policy in the Second Half of the 1980s." *Medical Care Review* 44 (Spring 1987): 65–88.

Physician Payment Review Commission (1989). *Annual Report to Congress.* Washington, D.C.: U.S. Government Printing Office.

Rovner, Julie (1989a). "Doctor Bills Are Next Target for Cost-Control Efforts." *Congressional Quarterly Weekly Report* 47 (February 25, 1989): 386–92.

Rovner, Julie (1989b). "Ways and Means OKs Overhaul of Medicare Payment Plan." *Congressional Quarterly Weekly Report* 47 (July 1, 1989): 1626–28.

Rovner, Julie (1989c). "Congress Agrees to Overhaul Medicare's Doctor Payments." *Congressional Quarterly Weekly Report* 47 (November 25, 1989): 3240–41.

Selected Bibliography

Aaron, H. J. and W. B. Schwartz. *The Painful Prescription: Rationing Health Care.* Washington, D.C.: Brookings Institution, 1984.

American Medical Association, Center for Health Policy Research. *Socioeconomic Characteristics of Medical Practice.* Chicago: American Medical Association, 1987.

Bendiner, R. *Obstacle Course on Capitol Hill.* New York: McGraw-Hill, 1965.

Eastaugh, S. *Medical Economics and Health Finance.* Dover, Mass.: Auburn House, 1981.

Eastaugh, S. *Financing Health Care: Economic Efficiency and Equity.* Dover, Mass.: Auburn House, 1987.

Eisenberg, J. M. *Doctor's Decisions and the Cost of Medical Care.* Ann Arbor, Mich.: Health Administration Press Perspectives, 1986.

Freidson, E., ed. *The Professions and Their Prospects.* Beverly Hills, Calif.: Sage, 1973.

Hadley, J. and R. A. Berenson. "Seeking the Just Price: Constructing Relative Value Scales and Fee Schedules." *Annals of Internal Medicine* 106 (1987): 461–66.

Holahan, J. F., and L. M. Etheredge, eds. *Medicare Physician Payment Reform—Issues and Options.* Washington, D.C.: Urban Institute Press, 1986.

Hsaio, W. C. et al. "Estimating Physicians' Work for a Resource-Based Relative-Value Scale." *New England Journal of Medicine* 319 (1988): 835–41.

Hsaio, W. C. et al. "Resource-Based Relative Values." *Journal of the American Medical Association* 260 (1988): 2347–53.

Hsaio, W. C. "Results and Policy Implications of the Resource-Based Relative Value Study." *New England Journal of Medicine* 319 (1988): 881–88.

Iglehart, J. K. "Medicare Begins Prospective Payment of Hospitals." *New England Journal of Medicine* 308 (1983): 1428–32.

Jencks, S. F., and A. Dobson. "Strategies for Reforming Medicare's Physician Payments." *New England Journal of Medicine* 312 (1985): 1492–99.

Langwell, K. M. and L. M. Nelson. "Physician Payment Systems: A Review of History, Alternatives and Evidence." *Medical Care Review* 43 (1986): 5–58.

Mitchell, J. "Physician DRGs." *New England Journal of Medicine* 313 (1985): 670–75.

President's Commission for the Study of Ethical Problems in Medicine and Biomedical and Behavioral Research. *Securing Access to Health Care: The Ethical Implications of Differences in the Availability of Health Services*. Washington, D.C.: U.S. Government Printing Office, 1983.

Reinhardt, U. "Resource Allocation in Health Care: The Allocation of Lifestyles to Providers." *Milbank Memorial Fund Quarterly* 65 (1987): 153–76.

Relman, A. "Salaried Physicians and Economic Incentives." *New England Journal of Medicine* 319 (1988): 784.

Roper, W. L. "Perspectives on Physician Payment Reform: The Resource Based Relative Value Scale in Context." *New England Journal of Medicine* 319 (1988): 865–67.

Ruby, G. "An Analysis of Methods to Reform Medicare Payment for Physician Services." *Inquiry* 24 (1987): 36–47.

Showstack, J. A. et al. "Fee-for-Service Physician Payment: Analysis of Current Methods and Their Development." *Inquiry* 16 (1979): 230.

Sloan, F. A., and J. W. Hay. "Medicare Pricing Mechanisms for Physician Services: An Overview of Alternative Approaches." *Medical Care Review* 43 (1986): 59–100.

Starr, P. *The Social Transformation of American Medicine*. New York: Basic Books, 1982.

U.S. Congress, Office of Technology Assessment. *Payment for Physician Services: Strategies for Medicare*. Washington, D.C.: U.S. Government Printing Office, 1986.

Index

About the Editor and Contributors

EDITOR

JONATHAN D. MORENO, Ph.D., was Associate Professor of Philosophy, of Health Care Sciences, and of Child Health and Development at The George Washington University. He is now Professor of Pediatrics and Director of the Division of Humanities in Medicine (Bioethics) at the SUNY Health Science Center at Brooklyn.

CONTRIBUTORS

MARY ANN BAILY, Ph.D., is Adjunct Associate Professor of Economics and of Health Care Sciences at The George Washington University.

JAMES BONANNO BAUTZ, M.D., J.D., is a Fellow in the Department of Health Care Sciences at The George Washington University.

ROBERT A. BERENSON, M.D., is Assistant Clinical Professor of Medicine at The George Washington University.

EDWARD BERKOWITZ, Ph.D., is Professor of History at The George Washington University.

JAMES F. CAWLEY, M.P.H., P.A.C., is Associate Professor of Health Care Sciences at The George Washington University.

GARY CRUM, Ph.D., is Associate Professor of Health Services Administration and of Health Care Sciences at The George Washington University.

ROBIN CURTIS was Morehead Scholar at The George Washington University and is now a journalist who plans to attend law school.

MOLLA DONALDSON, M.S., was Assistant Professor of Health Care Sciences at The George Washington University. She is now Senior Staff Officer at the Institute of Medicine, Washington, D.C.

STEVEN R. EASTAUGH, Sc.D., is Associate Professor of Health Services Administration and of Health Care Sciences at The George Washington University.

JACQUELINE J. GLOVER, Ph.D., is Assistant Professor of Health Care Sciences at The George Washington University.

JOHN F. HOADLEY, Ph.D., is Senior Research Associate in the National Health Policy Forum at The George Washington University.

JEAN JOHNSON, M.S.N., N.P.C., is Associate Professor of Health Care Sciences at The George Washington University.

JOHN E. OTT, M.D., is Professor of Health Care Sciences, of Child Health and Development, and of Health Services Administration at The George Washington University.

L. GREGORY PAWLSON, M.D., M.P.H., is Professor of Health Care Sciences, of Medicine, and of Health Services Administration at The George Washington University.

GAIL J. POVAR, M.D., is Associate Professor in the Department of Health Care Sciences at The George Washington University.

RICHARD K. RIEGELMAN, M.D., M.P.H., Ph.D., is Professor of Health Care Sciences, of Medicine, and of Health Services Administration at The George Washington University.

ROBERT S. SIEGEL, M.D., is Associate Professor of Medicine at The George Washington University.

JACK SUMMER, M.D., is Assistant Professor of Health Care Sciences and of Medicine at The George Washington University.

WENDY WOLFF, M.A., was a graduate student in the Department of History at The George Washington University. She is now Historical Editor at the U.S. Senate History Office.